普通高等教育“十一五”国家级规划教材

全国高等医药院校药学类实验双语教材

中药分析实验与指导（第2版）

Experiment and Guide for Pharmacology

主　编　刘丽芳
副主编　夏玉凤　杨　杰　许翔鸿　辛贵忠
编　者　（以姓氏笔画为序）
刘丽芳　许翔鸿　杨　杰
辛贵忠　夏玉凤

中国医药科技出版社

内 容 提 要

本教材是全国高等医药院校药学类实验双语教材之一。根据高等医药院校药学类中药分析课程的基本要求，结合实验教学经验及中药分析的发展现状，在第一版的基础上修订而成。全书共分为七章，包括生物碱类成分的分析，黄酮类成分的分析，醌类成分的分析，皂苷类成分的分析，挥发油类成分的分析，其他类成分的分析，中药制剂质量分析等内容。采用中英文对照，便于双语教学。适合高等教育药学类、中药学类专业师生使用。

图书在版编目（CIP）数据

中药分析实验与指导/刘丽芳主编．—2版．—北京：中国医药科技出版社，2015. 9
全国高等医药院校药学类实验双语教材
ISBN 978－7－5067－7747－6

Ⅰ. ①中…　Ⅱ. ①刘…　Ⅲ. ①中药材—药物分析—实验—医学院校—双语教学—教材　Ⅳ. ①R284. 1－33

中国版本图书馆 CIP 数据核字（2015）第 185597 号

美术编辑　陈君杞
版式设计　郭小平

出版　中国医药科技出版社
地址　北京市海淀区文慧园北路甲 22 号
邮编　100082
电话　发行：010－62227427　邮购：010－62236938
网址　www：cmstp. com
规格　787×1092mm 1/16
印张　9 3/4
字数　205 千字
初版　2003 年 8 月第 1 版
版次　2015 年 9 月第 2 版
印次　2023 年 12 月第 2 次印刷
印刷　三河市百盛印装有限公司
经销　全国各地新华书店
书号　ISBN 978－7－5067－7747－6
定价　29.00 元

序

教学是学校人才培养的中心环节，实验教学是这一环节的重要组成部分。《教育部、财政部关于“十二五”期间实施“高等学校本科教学质量与教学改革工程”的意见》要求进一步推进高等学校实验教学改革与创新，促进创新人才成长。《全国高等医药院校药学类实验双语教材》是中国药科大学自2005年以来坚持药学实践教学改革，突出提高学生动手能力、创新思维，通过承担教育部“世行贷款——21世纪初高等教育教学改革项目”等多项教改课题，逐步建设完善的一套与药学各专业学科理论课程紧密结合的高水平双语实验教材，也是普通高等教育“十一五”国家级规划教材。

本轮修订，适逢《全国高等医药院校药学类第四轮规划教材》及2015年版《中国药典》出版，整套教材的修订强调了与新版理论教材知识的结合，与2015年版《中国药典》、新版《药品质量管理规范》（GMP）等新颁布法典法规结合，为更好的服务于新时期高等院校药学教育与人才培养的需要，在上一版的基础上，进一步体现了各门实验课程自身独立性、系统性和科学性，又充分考虑到各门实验课程之间的联系与衔接，主要突出了以下特点。

1. 适应医药行业对人才的要求，体现行业特色 契合新时期药学人才需求的变化，使修订后的教材符合2015年版《中国药典》及新版GMP、新版GSP等国家标准、法规和规范以及新版国家执业药师资格考试大纲等行业最新要求。

2. 更新完善内容，打造教材精品 在上一轮教材基础上进一步优化、精炼和充实内容。紧密结合《全国高等医药院校药学类第四轮规划教材》，强调与实际需求相结合，进一步提高教材质量。

3. 坚持双语体系，强调素质培养 教材以实践教学为突破口，采用双语体系编写，有利于加快药学教育国际接轨，提高学生的科技英语水平，进一步提升学生整体素质。

《全国高等医药院校药学类实验双语教材》历经十年三轮建设，在各个时期广大编写教师的努力下，在广大使用教材师生的支持下日臻完善。本轮教材的出版，必将对推动新时期我国高等药学教育的发展产生积极而深远的影响。希望广大师生在教学实践中对本套教材提出宝贵意见，以便今后进一步修订完善，共同打造精品教材。

吴晓明

全国高等医药院校药学类规划教材常务编委会主任委员

二〇一五年八月

前　言

本版《中药分析实验与指导》实验双语教材是在全国高等医药院校药学类规划教材编委会的指导下，汲取上版教材的编写经验并结合实验教学实践的基础进行编写。本教材适合与《中药分析》、《中药制剂分析》等课程的课堂教学配套使用。编写过程中，在力求能够适应教育部建立有中国特色的药学高等教育体系新要求的基础上，对实验项目和内容进行了精心的选定和设计，进一步提高了教材的实用性和指导性。

本书共分八部分内容，即生物碱类成分的分析、黄酮类成分的分析、醌类成分的分析、皂苷类成分的分析、挥发油类成分的分析、其他类成分的分析、中药制剂质量分析和附录。本书有以下特点。

1. 内容较丰富，涵盖面广　包括了植物药各主要化学类型及不同剂型中药复方制剂质量分析等多方面的实验，共有实验 28 个，各校可根据具体条件和实际需要选择有关实验内容。

2. 强调实验方法的实用性和先进性　本教材的出版恰逢 2015 版《中国药典》的发行和实施，因此，所选的大部分实验都参考了最新版药典的方法和内容，并结合编委会成员的科研和教学经验，保证了实验内容的代表性、可操作性和重现性。

3. 强调现代分析方法的应用　本书所收载的实验分析方法主要为常用的薄层色谱法、高效液相色谱法、气相色谱法、紫外 – 可见分光光度法及液相色谱 – 质谱联用法等。

4. 强调对学生动手能力的培养　每个实验后有相关思考题和背景知识。为了便于学生参考和查阅，特别增加附录一章，所介绍内容包括常用中药质量分析方法、玻璃仪器的洗涤及各种洗液的配制法、常用溶剂的性质、色谱法预试中药化学成分和常用色谱显色剂及使用等。

由于编者的水平和经验有限，教材中可能存在疏漏、不足或不妥之处，敬请广大师生和读者提出宝贵意见，以便及时修正。

编　者

2015 年夏

Preface

This edition of Experiment and Guide for Analysis of Chinese Medicines is edited on the basis of our experience of the first bilingual edition and experimental teaching practices. It is suggested to be used together with such classroom teaching textbook as Analysis of Chinese Medicines and Analysis of Chinese medicine preparation. Throughout the compiling of this textbook, we strive to accord with the new requirements of Ministry of Education on the construction of pharmacy higher education system with Chinese characteristic and design most of the items and contents of experiment carefully to further improve the practicability and guidance.

The textbook is divided into 7 chapters, including analysis of alkaloids, flavonoids, quinones, saponins, volatile oil, other chemical constituents and Chinese medicine preparations as well as appendix. The characteristics of the book are as follows:

1. It has an abundant content and covers a wide range of aspects, involving the qualitative and quantitative of principal chemical components of plant medicines and diverse forms of Chinese medicine preparations, totally 28 experiments, providing a selection for different colleges considering their practical need and equipment available.

2. Focusing on the practicability and modernity of experimental method. The publication of the book is coincides with the issue and implement of Chinese Pharmacopoeia (2015 edition). Therefore, most of the experiments were designed according to the latest Pharmacopoeia, and combined with our research and teaching experiences. It guaranteed the representative, operability and repeatability of the content.

3. Emphasizing on the application of mordern analytical methods. Analytical methods recorded in the textbook are mainly thin layer chromatography, high - performance liquid chromatography, gas chromatography, ultraviolet - visible chromatography and liquid chromatography - mass spectrometry.

4. Putting emphasis on the cultivation of operation ability. There are background information and relative questions introduced at the end of each experiment. Especially an appendix was conceived to provide a reference easy to consult for students, consisting of quantitative methods of common Traditional Chinese Medicines (TCMs), wash-

ing procedure of glass apparatus and preparation of cleaning mixture, the property of commonly used solvents, thin layer chromatography conditions for TCMs with different components and the frequently used colorant in chromatography.

In condition with the limitation of our level and experiences, there must be some mistakes and defects in the textbook. Any criticism and advice are welcome.

The editorial board

Jul. 2015

目　录

第一章
生物碱类成分的分析

实验一　黄连中小檗碱的定性定量分析

【实验目的】

1. 熟悉离子对反相高效液相色谱法的原理和方法。

2. 掌握生物碱类样品制备方法和生物碱的通性。

【实验原理】

离子对色谱法测定的对象通常是常规反相色谱难以实施的分析对象，如极性的离子型化合物。它是将一种或几种与待分离组分分子电荷相反的离子，该离子具有大小不等的非极性基团或侧链，称为对离子或者反离子，加入到流动相中，使其与待测组分离子形成疏水型离子对化合物，再通过缓冲系统维持待测组分离子与反离子形成中性的离子对，通过控制待测组分离子在反相色谱中的保留行为，从而实现对离子型化合物反相分离的目的。

【实验器材】

1. 仪器　高效液相色谱仪－紫外检测器，ODS 反相色谱柱，微量进样器，展开缸等。

2. 试药与试剂　黄连药材，小檗碱对照品，高效硅胶 G 薄层板，色谱纯乙腈，磷酸二氢钾溶液，十二烷基硫酸钠，磷酸，环己烷，乙酸乙酯，异丙醇，甲醇，水，三乙胺。

【实验步骤】

1. 定性分析　称取黄连粉末 0. 25g，置于 50ml 的三角烧瓶中，加甲醇 25ml，水浴超声处理 30 分钟，滤过，取滤液作为供试品溶液。取黄连对照药材 0. 25g，同上法制成对照药材溶液。再取盐酸小檗碱对照品，加甲醇制成每 1ml 含 0. 5mg 的溶液，作为对照品溶液。吸取上述三种溶液各 1μl，分别点于同一高效硅胶 G 薄层板上，以环己烷: 乙酸乙酯: 异丙醇: 甲醇: 水: 三乙胺（3: 3. 5: 1: 1. 5: 0. 5: 1）作为展开剂，置用浓氨试液预饱和 20 分钟的展开缸内，展开，取出，晾干，置紫外光灯于 365nm 波长下检视。

黄连样品与对照药材色谱相应的位置上，显示 4 个以上相同颜色的荧光斑点；与小檗碱对照品色谱相应的位置上，显相同颜色的荧光斑点。

2. 定量分析

（1）色谱条件　色谱柱：十八烷基硅烷键合相硅胶色谱柱；流动相：乙腈：0.05mol/L 磷酸二氢钾溶液（50∶50）（每 100ml 中加十二烷基硫酸钠 0.4g，再以磷酸调节 pH 值为 4.0）为流动相；检测波长：345nm。

（2）对照品溶液的制备　取盐酸小檗碱对照品适量，精密称定，加甲醇制成浓度为 90.5μg/ml 的溶液。

（3）样品溶液的制备　黄连粉末，过二号筛，取上述粉末约 0.2g，精密称定，置具 100ml 塞锥形瓶中，精密加入甲醇－盐酸（100∶1）的混合溶液 50ml，密塞，称定重量，超声处理 30 分钟，放冷，再称定重量，用甲醇补足减失的重量，摇匀，滤过，精密量取续滤液 2ml，置 10ml 量瓶中，加甲醇至刻度，摇匀，滤过，取续滤液，即得。

（4）测定法　分别精密吸取小檗碱对照品溶液与黄连供试品溶液各 10μl，注入液相色谱仪，测定，以盐酸小檗碱对照品的峰面积为对照，通过外标一点法测定黄连中小檗碱的含量。

【实验记录】

1. 简要记录实验过程和出现的问题并讨论。

2. 计算小檗碱的含量，并根据文献资料讨论本实验结果中可能存在的其他黄连生物碱的峰面积及其保留时间。

【思考题】

1. 反相离子对色谱法需要加入何种类型的反离子？

2. 反相离子对色谱法适用于哪些类型化合物的含量测定？

【相关资料】

1. 药材来源　中药黄连为毛茛科植物黄连 *Coptis chinensis* Franch.、三角叶黄连 *Coptis deltoidea* C. Y. Cheng et Hsiao 或云连 *Coptis teeta* Wall. 的干燥根茎。以上三种分别习称“味连”、“雅连”、“云连”。

2. 化学成分　黄连含多种生物碱，主要含小檗碱，又称黄连素，约为 5%～8%，其次含黄连碱、表小檗碱、巴马亭、药根碱、非洲防己碱、甲基黄连碱等。本实验色谱条件下，表小檗碱、黄连碱、巴马汀、小檗碱色谱峰的相对保留时间如下：

黄连生物碱	相对保留时间
表小檗碱	0.71
黄连碱	0.78
巴马汀	0.91
小檗碱	1.00

小檗碱是一种常见的异喹啉生物碱，存在于小檗科等四个科十个属的许多植物中。

小檗碱是一种季铵生物碱，黄色针状晶体（乙醚）；熔点 145℃；溶于水，难溶于苯、乙醚和三氯甲烷。小檗碱盐在水中的溶解度较小，如盐酸盐为 1∶500，硫酸盐为1∶30。

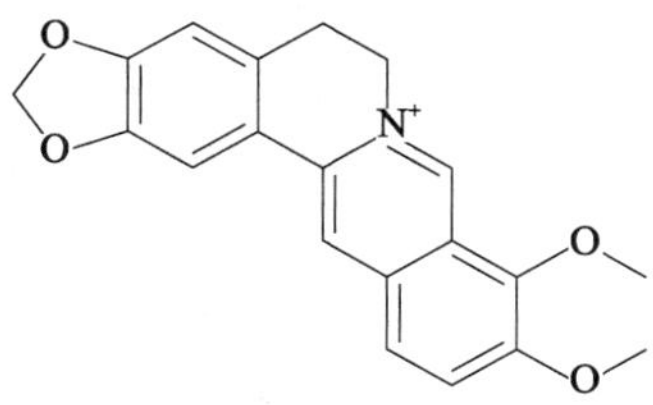

小檗碱

3. 功能与主治　黄连性寒味苦，归心、脾、胃、肝、胆、大肠经。具有清热燥湿，泻火解毒的作用。其中的小檗碱是常用的治疗肠道感染的植物抗生素。

Experiment 1　The Qualitative and Quantitative Analysis of Berberine in Coptidis Rhizoma

Purpose

1. To understand the principle and the method of ion pair reverse phase high performance liquid chromatography (HPLC) method.

2. To study the sample preparation method and the general character of the alkaloids.

Principle

Ion pair chromatography is a separate method for determination of a certain kind of analytes, such as the polar and ionic compounds, that are difficult using in the mode of regular reversed – phase chromatography. It is using one or more of so called "ion pair reagent", which generally possess a nonpolar side chain with opposite charge against the analytes. When added into the mobile phase, the ion pair reagent will combine analytes in a specified buffer solution and form hydrophobic complex, which could be retained in the reverse phase of the column, but the original analytes not. This method allows utilizing the traditional mode of reverse phase high performance liquid chromatography to separate the ionic compounds.

Conditions

1. Apparatus　High performance liquid chromatograph, octadecyltrimethoxysilane column, microsyringe and developing chamber.

2. Reagents and materials　Powder of Coptidis Rhizoma, berberine hydrochloride CRS (chemical reference substance), cyclohexane, ethyl acetate, isopropanol, methanol, triethylamine TLC plate of silica gel G, sodium dodecyl sulfate, sodium dodecyl sulfate, phosphoric acid, acetonitrile (chromatographic pure) and water.

Experimental Procedure

1. Qualitative analysis　To 0.25g of the powder of Coptidis Rhizoma, add 25ml of methanol, ultrasonicate for 30 minutes, filter and use the filtrate as the sample solution. Prepare a solution of 0. 25g of Coptidis Rhizoma reference drug in the same manner as the reference drug solution. Dissolve a quantity of berberine hydrochloride CRS in methanol to produce a solution containing 0. 5mg per ml as the reference solution. Use silica gel G as the coating substance and a mixture of cyclohexane, ethyl acetate, isopropanol, methanol, water and triethylamine (3∶3. 5∶1∶1. 5∶0. 5∶1) as the mobile phase. Apply separately to the plate 1μl of each of the above three solutions. After developing in a chamber pre – equilibrated with vapor of strong ammonia test solution (TS) for 20 minutes and removal of the plate, dry in air, examine under ultraviolet light at 365nm. The four fluorescent spots in the chromatogram will obtain with the sample solution correspond in position and color to the fluorescent spots in the chromatogram obtained with the reference drug solution, and one of which corresponds to the spot in the chromatogram obtained with the reference solution.

2. Quantitative analysis

(1) Chromatographic system and system suitability Use octadecylsilane bonded silica gel as the stationary phase and a mixture of acetonitrile and 0. 05mol/L solution of potassium dihydrogen phosphate (per 100ml add 0. 4g of sodium dodecyl sulfate, and adjust to pH 4. 0 by phosphoric acid) (50∶50) as the mobile phase. As detector a spectrophotometer set at 345nm. The number of theoretical plates of the column is not less than 5000, calculated with reference to the peak of berberine hydrochloride.

(2) Reference solution Weigh accurately a quantity of berberine hydrochloride CRS, dissolve in methanol to produce a solution containing 90. 5μg per ml as the reference solution.

(3) Test solution Weigh accurately 0. 2g of the powder (through No. 2 sieve) to a 100ml of stopper conical flask, add accurately 50ml of a mixture of methanol and hydrochloric acid (100∶1), weigh and ultrasonicate for 30 minutes, cool and weigh again, replenish the loss of the solvent with methanol, mix well and filter. Measure exactly 2ml of the successive filtrate to a 10ml volumetric flask, dilute with methanol to volume, mix well, filter and use the successive filtrate as the sample solution.

(4) Procedure Inject accurately 10μl of each of the reference solution and the sample solution, respectively, into the column for determination and calculate the content.

Experimental Records

1. Record the process, the phenomena and the problems of the experiment, and discuss them briefly.

2. Calculate the content of berberine, and according to the literature to discuss possible existing any other coptis alkaloids based on the HPLC results of this experiment and report their retention time and area of the peak.

Questions

1. What type of ion reagent should be added to the mobile phase in the ion pair reversed phase chromatography?

2. What type of compounds is suitable for the ion pair reversed phase chromatography?

Background Information

1. Origins Coptidis Rhizoma is called "huanglian" in China, whichis the dried rhizome of *Coptis chinensis* Franch., *Coptis deltoidea* C Y. Cheng et Hsiao or *Coptis teeta* Wall. (Fam. Ranunculaceae), commonly known as "Wei - lian", "Ya - lian" or "Yun - lian", respectively.

2. Chemical constituents Multiple alkanoids were isolated from Coptidis Rhizoma, such as berberine (about 5% ~ 8%), coptisine, epiberberine, palmatine, jatrorrhizine, columbamine and worenine.

In the conditions of this experiment, the relative retention times for berberine, coptisine, epiberberine and palmatine are as following:

Compound (peak)	Relative retention time
Epiberberine	0.71
Coptisine	0.78
Palmatine	0.91
Berberine	1.00

Berberine is an isoquinoline alkaloid in quartermary ammonium form. And it exists in many plants that belong to more than ten genera in four families, such as berberidaceae. In ether, berberine produces yellow needle crystal with melt point of 145℃. Berberine is soluble in water, insoluble in benzene, ether and chloroform. However, Berberine salt has small solubility in water, such as the hydrochloride is 1∶500 and the sulfate is 1∶30.

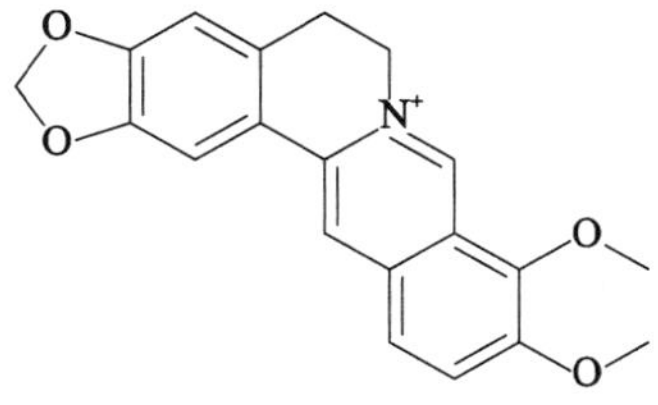

berberine

3. Actions and indications The property of Coptidis Rhizoma is *cold* and the flavor is bitter, and the meridian tropism is in heart, spleen, stomach, liver, gallbladder and large intestine meridians. The actions of this herb are to clear *heat* and dry dampness, purge *fire* and remove toxia. Berberine contained in this herb is an important plant antibiotics widely used for the treatment of intestinal infection.

实验二　附子中不同类型生物碱的定性定量分析

【实验目的】

1. 掌握反相高效液相色谱法测定生物碱的原理和方法。
2. 掌握反相高效液相色谱法常见流动相的使用注意事项。

【实验原理】

反相高效液相色谱属于反相液相色谱，即固定相的极性小于流动相的一种色谱分析方法。保留特性取决于分析物的疏水性，疏水性强的分析物保留强。现代高效液相色谱大多为是化学键合相，它对反相常见的极性流动相有良好的化学稳定性和热稳定性，色谱柱的柱效高，寿命长，重现性好，可分析的化合物多，几乎覆盖所有类型的有机化合物。

【实验器材】

1. 仪器　液相色谱仪－紫外检测器，ODS 反相色谱柱，微量进样器，展开缸等。

2. 试药与试剂　附子药材粉末，新乌头原碱对照品，苯甲酰乌头原碱对照品，苯甲酰次乌头原碱对照品，新乌头碱对照品、次乌头碱对照品、乌头碱对照品，异丙醇，二氯甲烷，乙醚，硅胶 G 薄层板正己烷，乙酸乙酯，甲醇，氨水，碘化铋钾试液，乙腈，四氢呋喃，醋酸铵，冰醋酸，色谱纯乙腈，水。

【实验步骤】

1. 定性分析　取苯甲酰新乌头原碱对照品、苯甲酰乌头原碱对照品、苯甲酰次乌头原碱对照品，加异丙醇－二氯甲烷（1∶1）混合溶液制成每 1ml 各含 1mg 的混合溶液，作为单酯型生物碱对照品溶液。取新乌头碱对照品、次乌头碱对照品、乌头碱对照品，加异丙醇－二氯甲烷（1∶1）混合溶液制成每 1ml 各含 1mg 的混合溶液，作为双酯型生物碱对照品溶液。取附子粉末 2g，加氨试液 3ml 润湿，加乙醚 25ml，超声处理 30 分钟，滤过。滤液挥干，残渣加二氯甲烷 0.5ml 使溶解，作为样品溶液。吸取供试品溶液和对照品溶液各 5～10μl，分别点于同一硅胶 G 薄层板上，以正己烷－乙酸乙酯－甲醇（6.4∶3.6∶1）为展开剂，置氨蒸气饱和 20 分钟的展开缸内，展开，取出，晾干，喷以稀碘化铋钾试液显色，日光下检视。

2. 定量分析

（1）色谱条件与系统适应性试验　色谱柱：C_{18} 柱；流动相：以乙腈－四氢呋喃（25∶15）为流动相 A，以 0.1mol/L 醋酸铵溶液（每 1000ml 加冰醋酸 0.5ml）为流动相 B，按下表中的规定进行梯度洗脱：

时间（分钟）	流动相 A（%）	流动相 B（%）
0～48	15→26	85→74
48～49	26→35	74→65
49～58	35	65
58～65	35→15	65→85

检测波长：235nm；理论板数按苯甲酰新乌头原碱峰计算应不低于3000。

（2）对照品溶液的制备　单酯型生物碱：取苯甲酰新乌头原碱对照品、苯甲酰乌头原碱对照品、苯甲酰次乌头原碱对照品适量，精密称定，加异丙醇－二氯甲烷（1∶1）混合溶液制成每1ml各含10μg的混合溶液，为单酯型生物碱对照溶液；双酯型生物碱：取新乌头碱对照品、次乌头碱对照品、乌头碱对照品适量，精密称定，加异丙醇二氯甲烷（1∶1）混合溶液制成每1ml各含5μg的混合溶液，为双酯型生物碱对照溶液。

（3）样品溶液的制备　取附子粉末（过三号筛）约2g，精密称定，置100ml具塞锥形瓶中，加氨试液3ml，精密加入异丙醇－乙酸乙酯（1∶1）混合溶液50ml，称定重量，在水温25℃以下超声处理30分钟，放冷，再称定重量，用异丙醇－乙酸乙酯（1∶1）混合溶液补足减失的重量，摇匀，滤过。精密量取续滤液25ml，40℃以下减压回收溶剂至干，残渣精密加入异丙醇－二氯甲烷（1∶1）混合溶液3ml溶解，滤过，取续滤液，即得。

（4）测定法　分别精密吸取对照品溶液与样品溶液各10μl，注入液相色谱仪，进行测定。以外标一点法计算上述六种生物碱的含量。

【实验记录】

1. 简要记录实验过程、实验现象及出现问题并讨论。

2. 计算六种生物碱的含量，并分别计算三种双酯型生物碱以及三种单酯型生物碱的总量。

【思考题】

1. 本实验中含量测定部分流动相B为何要使用醋酸铵并调节pH？

2. 附子的含量测定中为何要同时测定单酯型和双酯型生物碱的含量？

【相关资料】

1. 药材来源　附子为毛茛科植物乌头 *Aconitum carmichaelii* Debx的子根的加工品。经加工炮制为盐附子、黑附子（黑顺片）、白附片、淡附片、炮附片等。

2. 化学成分　乌头含乌头碱、新乌头碱以及次乌头碱等双酯型乌头生物碱。在乌头子根加工炮制为附子的过程中，双酯型乌头生物碱逐步水解为毒性较小的单酯型乌头生物碱，如苯甲酰乌头原碱、苯甲酰新乌头原碱、苯甲酰次乌头原碱等生物碱。单酯型乌头生物碱又可以水解为毒性更小的胺醇类碱，如乌头原碱、新乌头原碱、次乌头原碱。

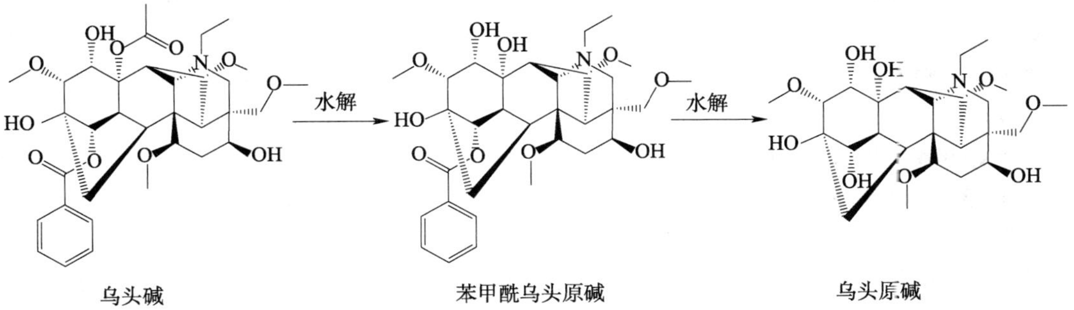

图1－1　乌头碱加工炮制过程中的水解反应

3. 功能与主治 附子性大热，味辛、甘，有毒。归心、肾、脾经。属于温里药，具回阳救逆，补火助阳，散寒除湿的功效，是经方四逆汤的君药及主要成分，为中药“回阳救逆第一品”。

Experiment 2 The Qualitative and Quantitative Analysis of Different Types of Aconite Alkaloids in Aconiti Lateralis Radix Praeparata

Purpose

1. To understand how the reversed – phase high performance liquid chromatography method to determine alkaloids and what the principle is.

2. To understand the characters of mobile phase which commonly used in reverse phase high performance liquid chromatography (RP – HPLC) and what should be to pay more attentions.

Principle

RP – HPLC is a type of reversed phase liquid chromatography which is defined as the polarity of the stationary phase is less than the mobile phase in a certain chromatographic system. The retention property of an analyte depends on its hydrophobicity that more strongly hydrophobic an analyte has, the more retentive the analyte is. Mobile phase in the modern HPLC generally is using so called “chemically bonded phase”. For most of the mobile phase being used in the RP – HPLC, chemically bonded phase possesses good chemical stability, as well as the thermal stability. Except above, it also represents an advantage of high column efficiency, long column life, and good reproducibility. It also provides possible to analyze more compounds that almost covers all types of organic compounds.

Conditions

1. Apparatus HPLC instrument, octadecyltrimethoxysilane column, microsyringe and developing chamber.

2. Reagents and materials Powder of Aconiti Lateralis Radix Praeparata, mesaconine CRS, hypaconitine CRS, aconitine CRS, benzoylmesaconine CRS, benzoylaconitine CRS and benzoylhypaconitine CRS, isopropanol, dichloromethane, tetrahydrofuran, ammonium acetate, glacial acetic acid, TLC plate of silica gel G, acetonitrile (chromatographic pure) and water.

Experimental Procedure

1. Qualitative analysis Macerate 2g of the powder with 3ml of ammonia test solution, add 25ml of ether, ultrasonicate for 30minutes and filter, evaporate the filtrate to dryness and dissolve in 0.5ml of dichloromethane as the test solution. Monoester – alkaloids: Dissolve benzoylmesaconine CRS, benzoylaconitine CRS and benzoylhypaconitine CRS and in a mixture of isopropanol and dichloromethane (1∶1) to produce a mixture containing 1mg of each per ml as the reference solution. Diester - alkaioids: Dissolve a quantity of mesaconine CRS, hypaconitine CRS and aconitine CRS in a mixture of isopropanol and dichloromethane (1:1) to produce a mixture containing 1mg of each per ml as the reference solution. Use silica gel G as the coating substance and a mixture of n - hexane, ethyl acetate and methanol (6.4:3.6:1) as the mobile phase. Apply separately to the plate 5 ~ 10μl of each of the sample solution and the reference solutions. After developing in a chamber pre equilibrated with ammonia vapor for 20 minutes and removal of the plate, dry in air, spray with dilute potassium iodobismuthate test solution and examine in day light.

2. Quantitative analysis

(1) Chromatographic system and system suitability Use octadecylsilane bonded silica gel as the stationary phase and a mixture of acetonitrile and tetrahydrofuran (25:15) as the mobile phase A, 0.1mol/L solution of ammonium acetate (add 0.5ml of glacial acetic acid per 1000ml) as the mobile phase B, elute in gradient as the following:

Time (min)	Mobile phase A (%)	Mobile phase B (%)
0 ~ 48	15→26	85→74
48 ~ 49	26→35	74→65
49 ~ 58	35	65
58 ~ 65	35→15	65→85

As detector a spectrophotometer set at 235nm. The number of theoretical plates of the column is not less than 3000, calculated with reference to the peak of benzoylme-saconine.

(2) Reference solution

Monoester - alkaloids: Dissolve benzoylmesaconine CRS, benzoylaconitine CRS and benzoylhypaconitine CRS in a mixture of isopropanol and dichloromethane (1:1) to produce a mixture containing 10μg of each per ml.

Diester - alkaioids: Weigh accurately mesaconine CRS, hypaconitine CRS and aconitine CRS respectively, dissolve in a mixture of isopropanol and dichloromethane (1:1) to produce a mixture containing 5μg of each per ml.

(3) Test solution Weigh accurately 2g of the powder (through No. 3 sieve) to a stopper conical flask, accurately add 3ml of ammonia test solution and 50ml of a mixture of isopropanol and ethyl acetate (1:1) and weigh. Ultrasonicate in water temperature below 30℃ for 30minutes, cool and weigh again, replenish the loss of solvent with the mixture of isopropanol and ethyl acetate (1:1) and mix well. Measure accurately 25ml of the successive filtrate and evaporate it to dryness in vacuum below 40℃. Dissolve exactly the residue in 3ml of a mixture of isopropanol and dichloromethane (1:1), mix well, filter and use the filtrate as the sample solution.

(4) Procedure Inject accurately 10μl of each of the reference solution and the test solution, respectively, into the column for determination and calculate the content.

Experimental Records

1. Record the process, the phenomena and the problems of the experiment, and discuss them briefly.

2. Calculate the content of six aconite alkaloids, and the sum of monoester type and diester type of aconite alkaloids respectively.

Questions

1. Why does the mobile phase B need to use ammonium acetate and adjust pH in the part "Quantitative anlysis" of this experiment?

2. Why need to simultaneously determine the monoester type and the diester type of aconite alkaloids?

Background Information

1. Origins Aconiti Lateralis Radix Praeparata also is called Fuzi in China, which is the processed daughter root of *Aconitum carmichaeli* Debx. (Fam. Ranunculaceae). It can be processed as Yanfuzi, Heifuzi (Heishunpian), Baifuzi, Danfuzi and Paofupian.

2. Chemical constituents The daughter root of *Aconitum carmichaeli* contain diester type alkaloids of aconitine, mesaconitine, hypaconitine etc., that are gradually hydrolyzed to less toxic monotype alkaloids, such as benzoylaconine, benzoylmesaconine, benzoylhypaconine in the process of Fuzi. The monotype alkaloids are further hydrolyzed into amino alcohols type alkaloids such as aconine, mesaconin and hypaconine, which are less more toxic.

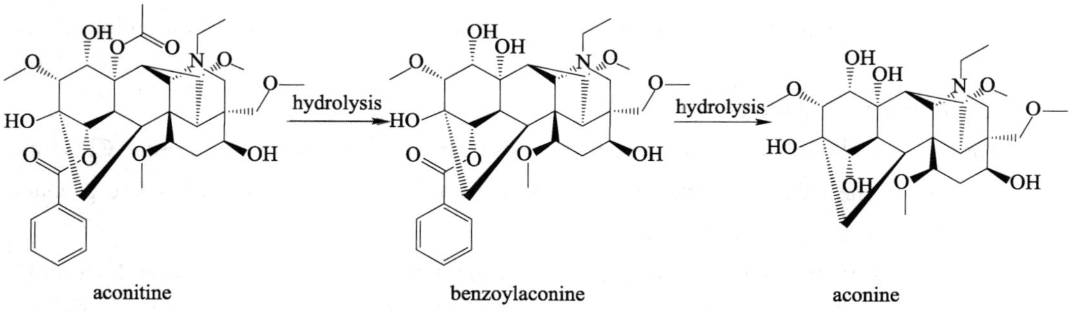

Figl -1: The hydrolysis reaction of aconitine in the process of Aconiti Lateralis Radix Praeparata

3. Actions and indications The property of Fuzi is highly hot and the flavor is pungent and sweet. It is toxic, and the meridian tropism is in heart, kidney and spleen meridians. Fuzi is a Chinese herb for inner - warming and with functions of restore Yang to save from collapse, tonify fire and assist Yang, dissipate cold and relieve pain. Fuzi is the main composition and the principal drug of "Sini Decoction" which recorded in "Shanghanlun", an ancient Chinese medical book means "treatise on febrile diseases". It is the first drug in the function of "rescuing from collapse by restoring Yang" in traditional Chinese drugs.

实验三　洋金花中阿托品类生物碱的定性定量分析

【实验目的】

1. 熟悉离子对反相高效液相色谱法的原理和方法。
2. 掌握生物碱类样品制备方法和生物碱的通性。

【实验原理】

同本章实验一。

【实验器材】

1. 仪器　高效液相色谱仪，紫外检测器，ODS色谱柱，微量进样器，展开缸等。

2. 试药与试剂　洋金花药材粉末，硫酸阿托品对照品、氢溴酸东莨菪碱对照品，甲醇，氨水，三氯甲烷，乙酸乙酯，甲醇，碘化铋钾试液，硅胶G薄层板，磷酸钠，磷酸，十二烷基硫酸钠，色谱纯乙腈，水。

【实验步骤】

1. 定性分析　取硫酸阿托品对照品、氢溴酸东莨菪碱对照品，加甲醇制成每1ml各含4mg的混合溶液，作为对照品溶液。取洋金花粉末1g，加浓氨试液1ml，混匀，加三氯甲烷25ml，摇匀，放置过夜，滤过，滤液蒸干，残渣加三氯甲烷1ml使溶解，作为供试品溶液。吸取对照品溶液与样品溶液各10μl，分别点于同一硅胶G薄层板上，以乙酸乙酯－甲醇－浓氨试液（17∶2∶1）为展开剂，展开，取出，晾干，喷以稀碘化铋钾试液显色。

2. 定量分析

（1）色谱条件与系统适应性试验　色谱柱：C_{18}柱；流动相：乙腈－0.07mol/L磷酸钠溶液（含0.0175mol/L十二烷基硫酸钠，用磷酸调节pH值至6.0）（50∶100）；检测波长：216nm。理论板数按氢溴酸东莨菪碱峰计算应不低于3000。

（2）对照品溶液的制备　精密称取氢溴酸东莨菪碱对照品适量，加流动相溶解并制成每1ml含0.5mg的溶液；东莨菪碱与氢溴酸东莨菪碱之间的换算公式：东莨菪碱重量＝氢溴酸东莨菪碱/1.445。

（3）样品溶液的制备　取过三号筛的洋金花粉末约1g，精密称定，置100ml的锥形瓶中，加入2mol/L盐酸溶液10ml，超声处理30分钟，放冷，滤过，滤渣和滤器用2mol/L盐酸溶液10ml分数次洗涤，合并滤液和洗液，用浓氨试液调节pH值至9，用三氯甲烷振摇提取4次，每次10ml，合并三氯甲烷液，回收溶剂至干，残渣用流动相溶解并转移至5ml量瓶中，稀释至刻度，摇匀。

（4）测定法　分别精密吸取对照品溶液与供试品溶液各10μl，注入液相色谱仪，测定，用外标一点法进行定量分析。

【实验记录】

1. 简要记录实验过程、实验现象及出现的问题并讨论。
2. 计算东莨菪碱的含量，并比对其他实验小组的结果，计算相对平均偏差。

【思考题】

1. 本实验中含量测定部分流动相中为何要使用十二烷基硫酸钠？

2. 本实验中样品溶液制备中为何要使用酸水提取？又为何用氨水碱化用三氯甲烷萃取？

【相关资料】

1. 药材来源 洋金花的基原为茄科植物白花曼陀罗 *Darura metel* Ld. 的干燥花。

2. 化学成分 洋金花含有莨菪烷类生物碱，包括莨菪碱（hyoscyamine），东莨菪碱（scopolamine），阿托品（atropine）等，该类成分既是洋金花的有效成分又是毒性成分，其含量必须严格控制，符合相关法典的监管要求。

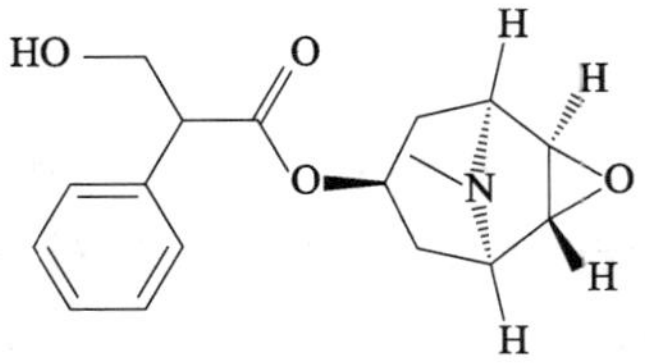

东莨菪碱

3. 功能与主治 洋金花性温味辛，有毒，归心、肺、脾经。具有平喘止咳，解痉定痛的功效。临床上用于哮喘咳嗽，脘腹冷痛，风湿痹痛，小儿慢惊。

Experiment 3 The Qualitative and Quantitative Analysis of Tropane Alkaloids in Daturae Flos

Purpose

1. To understand the principle and the method of ion pair reverse phase high performance liquid chromatography method.

2. To study the sample preparation method and the general character of the alkaloids.

Principle

Described as the same as the Experiment 1 of this chapter.

Conditions

1. Apparatus HPLC instrument, octadecyltrimethoxysilane column, microsyringe and developing chamber.

2. Reagents and materials Powder of Daturae Flos, chloroform, methanol, atropine sulfate CRS, scopolamine hydrobromide, ethyl acetate, ammonia, iodobismuthate test solution, TLC plate of silica gel G, sodium phosphate, sodium dodecyl sulfonate, phosphoric acid, acetonitrile (chromatographic pure) and water.

Experimental Procedure

1. Qualitative analysis To 1g of the powder add 1ml of concentrated ammonia test solution, mix well, add 25ml of chloroform, stir well. Allow to stand overnight, filter, evaporate the filtrate to dryness. Dissolve the residue in 1ml of chloroform, use the solution as the test solution. Dissolve a quantity of atropine sulfate CRS and scopolamine hydrobromide CRS in methanol to produce a solution containing 4mg of each per ml as the reference solution. Use silica gel G as the coating substance and a mixture of ethyl acetate, methanol and concentrated ammonia test solution (17:2:1) as the mobile phase. Apply 10μl of each of the two solutions to the plate. After developing and removal of the plate, dry in air, spray with dilute potassium iodobismuthate test solution. Compare the spots in the chromatogram obtained with the sample solution correspond in position and color to those obtained with the reference solution.

2. Quantitative analysis

(1) Chromatographic system and system suitability　Use octadecylsilane bonded silica gel as the stationary phase and a mixture of acetonitrile and a 0.07mol/L sodium phosphate buffer (containing 0.0175mol/L sodium dodecyl sulfonate, adjust pH to 6.0 with phosphoric acid) (50:100) as the mobile phase. As detector a spectrophotometer set at 216nm. The number of theoretical plates of the column is not less than 3000, calculated with reference to the peak of scopolamine hydrobromide.

(2) Reference solution　Weigh accurately a quantity of scopolamine hydrobromide CRS and dissolve in the mobile phase to produce a solution of 0.5mg per ml (The weight of scopolamine equals to that of scopolamine hydrobromide divided by 1.445).

(3) Test solution　Weigh accurately 1g of the powder (through No. 3 sieve) in a conical flask, add 10ml of 2mol/L hydrochloric acid, and ultrasonicate for 30 minutes, cool and filter, wash the residue and the filter with 10ml of 2mol/L hydrochloric acid in portions, combine the filtrates and washings, adjust pH to 9.0 with concentrated ammonia test solution, extract by shaking with four 10ml quantities of chloroform, combine the chloroform extracts, recover chloroform to dryness. Dissolve the residue in the mobile phase, transfer to a 5ml volumetric flask, dilute to volume and mix well.

(4) Procedure　Inject accurately 10μl of each of the reference solution and the sample solution, respectively, into the column for determination and calculate the content.

Experimental Records

1. Record the process, the phenomena and the problems of the experiment, and discuss them briefly.

2. Calculate the content of scopolamine, and calculate the relative standard deviation (RSD) by comparing with the results of other groups.

Questions

1. Why the mobile phase use sodium dodecyl sulfate in this experiment?

2. Why need to use acid water for extraction in the sample preparations? And on the other hand, why alkalizing the sample in the next step by ammonia and using chloroform for extraction?

Background Information

1. Origins　Daturae Flos is also called yangjinhua in China, which is derived from dried flowers of *Datura metel* L. (Fam. Solanaceae).

2. Chemical constituents　Daturae Flos contains tropane alkaloids, including hyoscyamine, scopolamine, atropine, etc. Tropane alkaloids are the active and the toxic components contained in this crude drug. The content of tropane alkaloids in this drug must be in control for clinical use, and their contents must meet the regulation requirements.

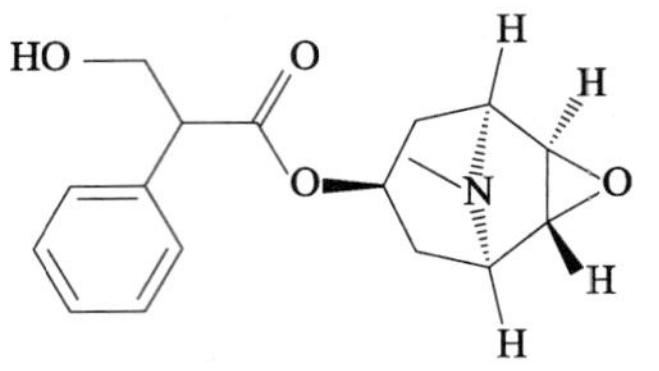

scopolamine

3. Actions and indications Daturae Flos is a toxic traditional Chinese drug, its property is *warm* and the flavor is pungent, and the meridian tropism is in lung and liver meridians. It is clinically used for asthma, cough, cold pain in the epigastrium and abdomen, painful impediment caused by *wind dampness* and chronic infantile convulsion.

实验四　高效液相色谱–质谱联用法测定千里光中阿多尼弗林碱的含量

【实验目的】

1. 掌握高效液相色谱–质谱联用法的基本原理。
2. 掌握通过内标物法定量的计算方法。

【实验原理】

高效液相色谱–质谱联用法是将以分离技术见长的色谱方法与物质定性定量见长的质谱方法相结合的一项分析技术。样品首先在高效液相色谱上完成分离，然后通过高效液相色谱与质谱的接口模块——离子源，将样品转换为质谱可以接受的形式。通常高效液相色谱质谱法常用的离子源为电喷雾离子源（Electrospray Ionization，ESI），它是通过对样品液流的雾化，在高压电场的库仑力与干燥气的双重作用下，气化液滴并逐步脱溶剂，完成样品分子的离子化，并将离子化后的样品送入下游的质量分析器进行分析，最终完成定性与定量。

【实验器材】

1. 仪器　液相色谱仪–质谱检测器，ODS反相色谱柱，微量进样器等。

2. 试药与试剂　千里光药材粉末，阿多尼弗林碱对照品，野百合碱对照品，甲酸，色谱纯乙腈，超纯水。

【实验步骤】

1. 色谱和质谱条件与系统适应性试验　色谱柱：以十八烷基硅烷键合硅胶色谱柱；流动相：以乙腈–0.5%甲酸溶液（7∶93）为流动相。检测器为单级四极杆质谱检测器；离子化方式为电喷雾离子化（ESI），正离子模式；数据采集模式：选择离子监测（Selected Ion Monitoring，SIM）方式，对质荷比（m/z）为366离子进行检测。

2. 对照品溶液的制备　取阿多尼弗林碱对照品适量，精密称定，加0.5%甲酸溶液制成每1ml含0.1μg的溶液，作为对照品溶液。

3. 内标溶液的制备 取野百合碱对照品适量，精密称定，加0.5%甲酸溶液制成每1ml含0.2μg的溶液，作为内标溶液。

4. 样品溶液的制备 取过三号筛的千里光粉末约0.2g，精密称定，置100ml具塞锥形瓶中，精密加入0.5%甲酸溶液50ml，称定重量，超声处理40分钟，放冷，再称定重量，用0.5%甲酸溶液补足减失的重量，摇匀，滤过，精密量取续滤液2ml，置5ml量瓶中，精密加入内标溶液1ml，加0.5%甲酸溶液至刻度，摇匀。

5. 校正因子测定 精密量取对照品溶液2ml，置5ml量瓶中，精密加入内标溶液1ml，加0.5%甲酸溶液至刻度，摇匀，吸取2μl，注入液相色谱－质谱联用仪，计算校正因子。

6. 测定法 分别精密吸取对照品溶液与供试品溶液各10μl，注入液相色谱仪，测定，以内标法计算阿多尼弗林碱的含量。

【实验记录】

1. 简要记录实验过程，实验现象及出现问题并讨论。

2. 计算阿多尼弗林碱/野百合碱的校正因子，并通过该校正因子计算阿多尼弗林碱的含量。

【思考题】

1. 本实验中色谱条件中，测定的对象为生物碱，但流动相中为何要使用甲酸？

2. 使用内标法进行含量测定有哪些优点和缺点？

【相关资料】

1. 药材来源 千里光为菊科植物千里光 *Senecio scandens* Buch. －Ham. 的干燥地上部分。

2. 化学成分 千里光全草含大量的毛茛黄素、菊黄质；此外还含有黄酮类、生物碱类等成分。其中生物碱类成分的结构类型为吡咯里西啶类生物碱（pyrrolizidine alkaloids，PAs），PAs是已知的植物肝脏毒性成分之一，它是千里光的毒性成分，必须加以监控。

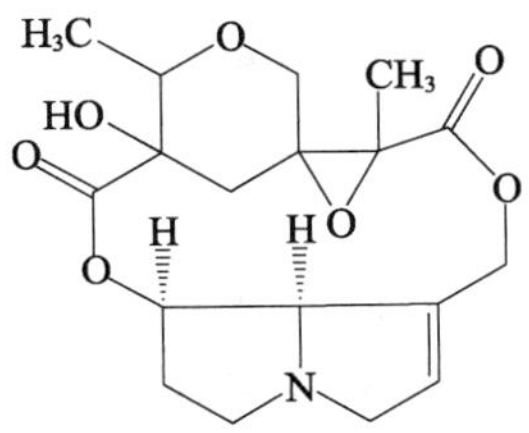

阿多尼弗林碱

3. 功效 千里光性寒，味苦，归肺、肝经。具有清热，解毒，杀虫，明目的功效。

（许翔鸿）

Experiment 4 The Determination of Adonifoline in Senecionis Scandentis Herba by HPLC – MS

Purpose

1. To understand the basic principle of high performance liquid chromatography coupled with mass spectrometry (HPLC/MS).

2. To master the quantitative method by using internal standard.

Principle

HPLC – MS is an analytical technique that combined in liquid chromatography (LC) which good at separating with mass spectrometry (MS) that good at qualitative. First of all, the analytes is separated by LC, and then the analytes pass the interface which is between LC and MS called ion source, and then the analytes are ionized to ion that can be analyzed by the mass spectrometer. The ion source for HPLC – MS usually is electrospray ion source (ESI). The mechanism of ionization is that the ESI ion source sprays the LC stream to form charged liquid drops, which gradually evaporate by dry gas. Finally the coulomb explosion is produced to ionize the analytes. The ionized sample is induced into the mass analyzer for determining to produce the mass data that can qualify and quantify the sample.

Conditions

1. Apparatus HPLC – MS instrument and C_{18} column.

2. Reagents and materials Senecionis Scandentis Herba, adonifoline CRS, monocrotaline CRS, formic acid, acetonitrile (chromatographic pure) and ultra pure water.

Experimental Procedure

1. Chromatographic and spectrometric system and system suitability Use octadecylsilane bonded silica gel as the stationary phase and a mixture of acetonitrile and 0.5% formic acid solution (7∶93) as the mobile phase. As detector a single quadrupole mass spectrometry with an ESI positive ion interface set at m/z 366 in a selective ion monitoring (SIM) mode. The number of theoretical plates of the column is not less than 8000, calculated with reference to the peak of adonifoline.

2. Reference solution Dissolve a quantity of adonifoline CRS, accurately weighed, in 0.5% formic acid to prepare a solution containing 0.1μg per ml as the reference solution.

3. Internal standard solution Dissolve a quantityof monocrotaline CRS, accurately weighed, in 0.5% formic acid to prepare a solution containing 0.2μg per ml as a internal standard solution.

4. Correction factor Measure accurately 2ml of the reference solution and 1ml of the internal standard solution to a 5ml volumetric flask, dilute with 0.5% formic acid to volume, and mix well. Inject accurately 2μg of the solution into column and calculate the correction factor for adonifoline.

5. Test solution Weigh accurately 0.2g of the powder (through No. 3 sieve) in a stoppered conical flask, add 50ml of 0.5% formic acid, and weigh, ultrasonicate for 40 minutes, allow to cool and weigh again, replenish the loss of weight with 0.5% formic acid, mix well and filter. Measure accurately 2ml of the successive filtrate and 1ml of the internal standard solution in a 5ml volumetric flask and dilute with 0.5% formic acid to volume and mix well as the test solution.

6. Procedure Inject accurately 2μl of the sample solution into column and calculate the content.

Experimental Records

1. Record the process, the phenomena and the problems of the experiment, and discuss them briefly.

2. Calculate the correction factor of adonifoline with monocrotaline, and calculate the content of adonifoline according the correction factor.

Questions

1. Why we use formic acid solution as the mobile phase to determine the content of alkaloids in this experiment?

2. What advantages and disadvantages in the content determination by using the internal standard method?

Background Information

1. Origins Senecionis Scandentis Herba is also called "Qianliguang" in China, which is the dried aerial part of *Senecio scandenes* Buch. – Ham. (Fam. Compositae).

2. Chemical constituents Senecionis Scandentis Herba contains a mass of flavoxanthin and chrysanthemaxanthin. Except above, it also contains flavonoids and alkaloids. The structure of alkaloids in Qianliguang is pyrrolizidine alkaloids (PAs). PAs is known as the compound of hepatotoxicity, and must to be controlled for clinical use. China pharmacopoeia specifiesthe content of adonifoline is not more than 0.004 per cent in the dried crude drug.

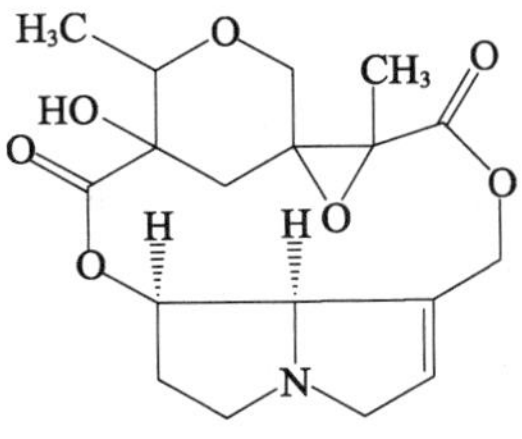

adonifoline

3. Actions and indications The property of qianliguang is cold, and its flavor is bitter, and the meridians tropism is in lung and liver meridians. The functions are to clear heat and remove toxin, improve vision, and drain dampness.

(Xianghong Xu)

第二章
黄酮类成分的分析

实验一　槐花中黄酮类成分的定性定量分析

【实验目的】

1. 掌握黄酮类成分的性质及其定性定量方法。
2. 掌握薄层色谱法的操作技术及其在黄酮类成分定性中的应用。
3. 掌握紫外可见分光光度计的使用。

【实验原理】

1. 薄层色谱法的原理　薄层色谱法是一种用于分离混合物的色谱技术。薄层色谱在覆盖有很薄的一层吸附剂的玻璃板、塑料片或铝箔上进行。吸附剂又称为薄层色谱固定相，常为硅胶、氧化铝或纤维素。操作时先将待分离样品用毛细管点于板上，然后在密闭的层析缸中，用单一或混合溶剂作为流动相。由于吸附剂对不同组分具有不同的吸附能力，展开剂对不同组分也有不同的溶解、解吸能力，因此当展开剂不断展开，不同组分会在吸附剂和展开剂之间发生连续不断的吸附、解吸附，从而产生差速迁移得到分离。

薄层色谱中的 R_f值可作为定性鉴别的依据。应用 R_f定性，一般用待测化合物的纯品作对照，若样品中斑点的 R_f值与纯品 R_f值都相同，可推测两者为同一化合物。但在中药鉴定中也常用标准药材为对照品，用以鉴别药材的真伪。

黄酮类成分的薄层定性，一般采用吸附薄层，常用的吸附剂有硅胶与聚酰胺，硅胶分离黄酮成分遵循正相色谱规律，化合物极性越强，所需溶剂的极性越大。由于黄酮类成分大多具有紫外吸收，紫外灯下观察定位是黄酮类成分定性的最常用的方法，如再配合数种显色剂，就可以帮助鉴定各种类型的黄酮，还可以帮助鉴别药材品种。

2. 紫外可见分光光度法原理　紫外可见分光光度法是以紫外 - 可见光区的光谱作为光源，研究物质对光的吸收强度的方法。根据 Lambert - Beer 定律，物质的吸光度与物质的浓度成正比，从而实现对化学结构上具有共同特征的大类成分的定量。黄酮类化合物分子结构中多含有羰基和羟基等结构，这些结构可与金属盐类试剂如铝盐、铅盐等生成有色配合物，因而可以利用这一性质对药材中的总黄酮的含量进行测定。

【实验器材】

1. 仪器　紫外分光光度计，移液管，容量瓶，锥形瓶，量筒，三用紫外分析仪，水浴锅，索氏提取器，展开缸。

2. 试药与试剂　槐花药材，芦丁对照品，薄层硅胶G板，乙醇，盐酸，镁粉，甲醇，乙酸乙酯，水，10%三氯化铝乙醇溶液，氢氧化钠试液，10%硝酸铝溶液，5%亚硝酸钠溶液，乙醚。

【实验步骤】

1. 定性分析

（1）化学定性分析　取本品0.2g，加乙醇5ml，水浴温热5分钟，滤过。取滤液2ml，加镁粉少许，混匀，滴加盐酸数滴，即显樱红色。（检查黄酮）

（2）薄层色谱定性分析　取本品粉末约0.2g，加甲醇5ml，密塞，振摇10分钟，滤过，取滤液作为供试品溶液。另取芦丁对照品，加甲醇制成每1ml含4mg的溶液，作为对照品溶液。照薄层色谱法试验，吸取上述两种溶液各10μl，分别点于同一硅胶G薄层板上，以乙酸乙酯－甲醇－水（8∶1∶1）作为展开剂，展开，取出，晾干，喷以10%三氯化铝乙醇溶液，置紫外灯（365nm）下检视。供试品色谱中，在与对照品色谱相应的位置上，显相同颜色的荧光斑点。

2. 定量分析

（1）对照品溶液的制备　精密称取在120℃干燥至恒重的芦丁对照品50mg，置25ml量瓶中，加甲醇适量，置水浴上微热使溶解，放冷，加甲醇至刻度，摇匀。精密量取10ml，置100ml量瓶中，加水至刻度，摇匀，即得（每1ml中含无水芦丁0.2mg）。

（2）标准曲线的制备　精密量取对照品溶液1ml、2ml、3ml、4ml、5ml与6ml，分别置25ml量瓶中，各加水至6ml，加5%亚硝酸钠溶液1ml，混匀，放置6分钟，加10%硝酸铝溶液1ml，摇匀，放置6分钟，加氢氧化钠试液10ml，再加水至刻度，摇匀，放置15分钟，以相应试剂为空白，照紫外－可见分光光度法，在500nm波长处测定吸光度，以吸光度为纵坐标，浓度为横坐标，绘制标准曲线。

（3）测定法　取本品粗粉约1g，精密称定，置索氏提取器中，加乙醚适量，加热回流至提取液无色，放冷，弃去乙醚液。再加甲醇90ml，加热回流至提取液无色，转移至100ml量瓶中，用甲醇少量洗涤容器，洗液并入同一量瓶中，加甲醇至刻度，摇匀。精密量取10ml，置100ml量瓶中，加水至刻度，摇匀。精密量取3ml，置25ml量瓶中，照标准曲线制备项下的方法，自“加水至6ml”起，依法测定吸光度，从标准曲线上读出供试品溶液中含无水芦丁的重量（μg），计算，即得。

【实验记录】

1. 记录槐花提取液加盐酸，镁粉反应后的实验现象。
2. 绘制定性薄层图，记录芦丁在本实验的薄层色谱条件下的 R_f 值。
3. 绘制芦丁的标准曲线图。
4. 计算槐花中总黄酮的含量。

【思考题】

1. 为什么要取续滤液作为测定溶液？否则对测定结果有何影响？
2. 样品测定项下加石油醚回流的目的是什么？

【相关资料】

1. 药材来源 槐花（槐米）为豆科植物槐 *Sophora japonica* L. 的干燥花及花蕾。夏季花开放或花蕾形成时采收，及时干燥，除去枝、梗及杂质。前者习称“槐花”；后者习称“槐米”。

2. 化学成分 槐花（槐米）中主含芦丁（芸香苷），约占28%，其苷元为槲皮素；并含有桦皮醇、槐二醇、槐花米甲、乙、丙素等。

2015 版《中国药典》规定本品含芦丁，槐花不得少于 8.0%，槐米不得少于 20.0%（用紫外分光光度法）；另规定醇浸出物（30% 甲醇）槐花不得少于 37%，槐米不得少于 43%。

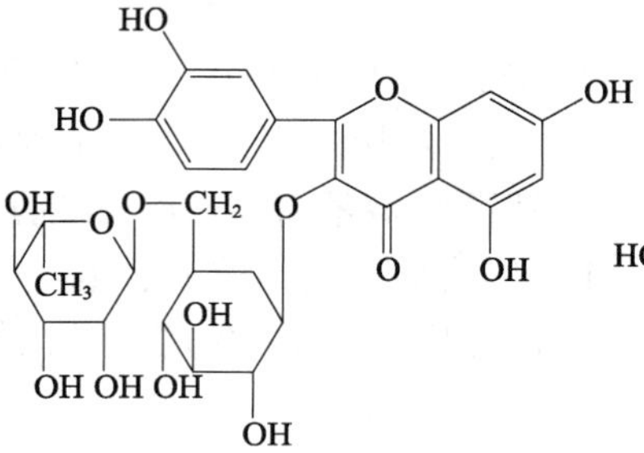

芦丁

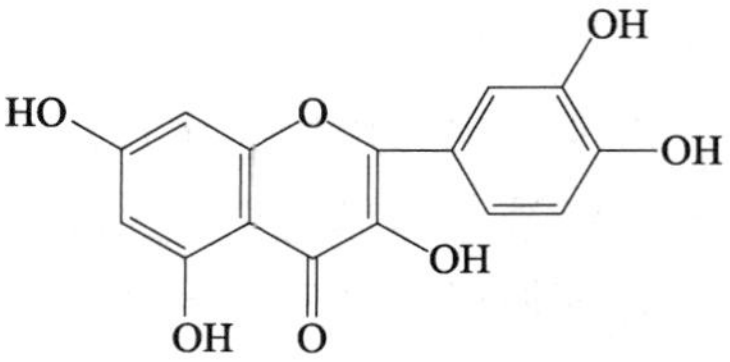

槲皮素

3. 理化性质

（1）芦丁（$C_{27}H_{30}O_{16}$，芸香苷）：系黄酮类化合物的糖苷，分子量为 610.51。浅黄色针状结晶（水），熔点 176 ~ 178℃，加热至 185 ~ 192℃ 成棕色，215℃ 时分解。$[\alpha]_D^{23}$ +13.82°（乙醇）。能溶于二甲基亚砜和吡啶，甲酰和碱液；微溶于乙醇，丙酮和乙酸乙酯，几乎不溶于水、三氯甲烷、乙醚、苯、二硫化碳和石油醚。UVλ_{Max}^{MeOH}nm：258、361。在 2% 稀酸下水解得苷元槲皮素。

（2）槲皮素（$C_{15}H_{10}O_7$）：分子量为 302.23。二水合物为黄色针状结晶（稀乙醇），在 95 ~ 97℃ 成为无水物，熔点 314℃（分解）。能溶于冷乙醇（1∶290），易溶于热乙醇（1∶23），可溶于甲醇、乙酸乙酯、冰醋酸、吡啶、丙酮等，不溶于水、苯、乙醚、三氯甲烷、石油醚等。UV λ_{Max}^{EtOH}nm：258（2.75）、375（2.75）。

4. 功效主治 具有凉血止血，清肝泻火的功效；用于便血，痔血，血痢，崩漏，吐血，衄血，肝热目赤，头痛眩晕。

Experiment 1 The Qualitative and Quantitative Analysis of Flavonoids in Sophorae Flos

Purpose

1. Comprehend the qualitative and quantitative analysis of flavonoids.

2. Comprehend the principle and operation of thin – layer chromatography in the analysis of flavonoids.

3. Comprehend the principle and operation of ultraviolet detector through this experiment.

Principle

1. Thin – layer chromatography Thin – layer chromatography (TLC) is a chromatography technique used to separate mixtures. TLC is performed on a sheet of glass, plastic, or aluminum foil, which is coated with a thin layer of adsorbent material, usually silica gel, aluminium oxide, or cellulose. This layer of adsorbent is known as the stationary phase. After the sample has been applied on the plate, a solvent or solvent mixture (known as the mobile phase) is drawn up the plate via capillary action. Different compounds in the sample mixture travel at different rates due to the differences in their attraction to the stationary phase and the differences in solubility in the solvent. Because different analytes ascend the TLC plate at different rates, separation is achieved.

After a separation is complete, individual compounds appear as spots separated vertically. Each spot has a retention factor (R_f) which is equal to the distance migrated over the total distance covered by the solvent. The R_f value can be used to identify compounds due to their uniqueness to each compound in the same condition. If the R_f value in our sample is the same as this of reference under the same condition, they might be the same compound. In addition, in the qualification of Traditional Chinese Medicine, the reference drug is commonly used.

As for flavonoids, silica gel and polyamide are usually used as the stationary phase. When silica is used as stationary phase, separation of compounds is based on the polarity of the compounds. The more polar compound has a stronger interaction with the silica and therefore, has a smaller R_f value. As flavonoids have good absorption under UV light, the spots of compounds can be seen by illuminating the plate with short – wave UV. A number of chemical stains can be used such as the solution of $AlCl_3$.

2. Ultraviolet – visible spectroscopy Ultraviolet – visible spectroscopy (UV – Vis) refers to absorption spectroscopy or reflectance spectroscopy in the ultraviolet – visible spectral region. This means it uses light in the visible and adjacent (near – UV) ranges. The absorption or reflectance in the visible range directly affects the perceived color of the chemicals involved. The Lambert – Beer law states that the absorbance of a solution is directly proportional to the concentration of the absorbing species in the solution and the path length. Thus, for a fixed path length, UV/V is spectroscopy can be used to determine the concentration of the absorber in a solution. As flavonoids contain many carbonyl and hydroxyl groups, they can react with many metal salts reagents such as aluminum, lead salts and generate colored complexes. Therefore, the content of total flavonoids can be determined by UV – Vis.

Conditions

1. Apparatus Ultraviolet detector, ultraviolet analyzer, Soxhlet's extractor, pipette, volumetric flask, conical flask, measuring cylinder, water bath and developing chamber.

2. Reagents and materials Sophorae flos, rutin, silica gel G, methanol, hydrochloric acid – magnesium powder, ethanol, ethyl acetate, water, 10% aluminum trichloride in ethanol, 5% sodium nitrate, sodium hydroxide solution, 10% aluminum nitrate.

Experimental Procedure

1. Qualitative analysis

(1) Chemical qualitative analysis To 0.2g of the powder with 5ml of ethanol, heat for 5 minutes and filter. To 1ml of the filtrate, add a small quantity of magnesium powder and 2 ~ 3 drops of hydrochloric acid, a cherry red colour is produced.

(2) TLC qualitative analysis Shake 0.2g of the powder with 5ml of methanol for 10 minutes, and filter, use the filtrate as the test solution. Dissolve a quantity of rutin CRS in methanol to produce a solution containing 4mg per ml as the reference solution. Carry out the method for thin layer chromatography, using silica gel G as the coating substance and a mixture of ethyl acetate, formic acid and water (8∶1∶1) as the mobile phase. Apply separately to the plate 10μl of each of the above two solutions. After developing and removal of the plate, dry in air, spray with a 1% aluminum chloride in ethanol. Examine under ultraviolet light at 365nm. A fluorescent spot in the chromatogram obtained with the test solution corresponds in position and color to the fluorescent spot obtained with the reference solution.

2. Quantitative Analysis

(1) Reference solution Weigh accurately 50mg of rutin CRS to a 25ml volumetric flask and dissolve with a quantity of methanol by warming gently on a water bath. Allow to cool, add methanol to volume and mix well. Measure accurately 10ml of the solution into a 100ml volumetric flask, dilute with water to volume and mix well (containing 0.2mg of anhydrous rutin per ml).

(2) Calibration standard Measure accurately 1ml, 2ml, 3ml, 4ml, 5ml and 6ml of the reference solution into a 25ml volumetric flask, respectively, add water to 6.0ml and add lml of a 5% solution of sodium nitrate, mix well. Allow to stand for 6 minutes, add 1ml of a 10% solution of aluminum nitrate, mix well, stand for 6 minutes again and add 10ml of sodium hydroxide TS, dilute with water to volume. Mix well and stand for 15 minutes. Carry out the method for ultraviolet spectrophotometry and colorimetry by using the corresponding solvent as a blank, immediately measure the absorbance at 500nm and plot the standard curve, using absorbance as ordinate and concentration as abscissa.

(3) Procedure Weigh accurately 1g of the coarse powder, to a Soxhlet's extractor, add a quantity of ether and heat under reflux until the extract colourless. Allow to cool, and discard ether extract. Add 90ml of methanol, heat under reflux until the extract colourless. Transfer the extract to a 100ml volumetric flask, wash the flask with a small quantity of methanol, combine the washings into the volumeric flask, add methanol to volume and mix well. Measure accurately 10ml to a 100ml volumetric flask, add water to volume and mix well. Transfer accurately 3ml of the solution to a 25ml volumetric flask, carry out the procedure as described under calibration standard, beginning at the words "add water to 6.0ml", Measure the absorbance, read out the weight of anhydrous rutin in the test solution from the standard curve, and calculate the content of $C_{27}H_{30}O_{16}$.

Experimental Records

1. Record the experimental phenomena after the hydrochloric acid magnesium powder was added into the extract.

2. Draw the TLC chromatogram and record the R_f value of rutin.

3. Plot the standard curve of rutin.

4. Calculate the content of total flavonoids in Sophorae Flos.

Questions

1. Why do we use successive filtrate as the test solution? What the results would be if not?

2. What is the purpose of refluxing with petroleum ether?

Background Information

1. Origins Sophorae Flos is the dried flower and flower bud of *Sophora japonica* L. (Fam. Leguminosae). It is collected in summer at flowering or when flower buds are forming, dried in time and removed from branch, pedicel and foreign matter. The former is known as "Huaihua", and the later "Huaimi".

2. Chemical constituents Rutin is a main compound in Sophorae Flos. Its content is up to 28% in Huaimi. Quercetin is the aglycone of rutin. Sophorae Flos also contains botulin, sophoradiol, sophorin A, B, C and so on.

In People's Republic of China Pharmacopoeia (2015 edition), it should contain not less than 8.0 per cent of anhydrous rutin ($C_{27}H_{30}O_{16}$) for Huaihua and not less than 20.0 per cent of anhydrous rutin ($C_{27}H_{30}O_{16}$) for Huaimi, calculated with reference to the dried drug.

It contains not less than 37.0 per cent of anhydrous rutin ($C_{27}H_{30}O_{16}$) for Huaihua and not less than 43.0 per cent of anhydrous rutin ($C_{27}H_{30}O_{16}$) for Huaimi, calculated with reference to the alcohol extract.

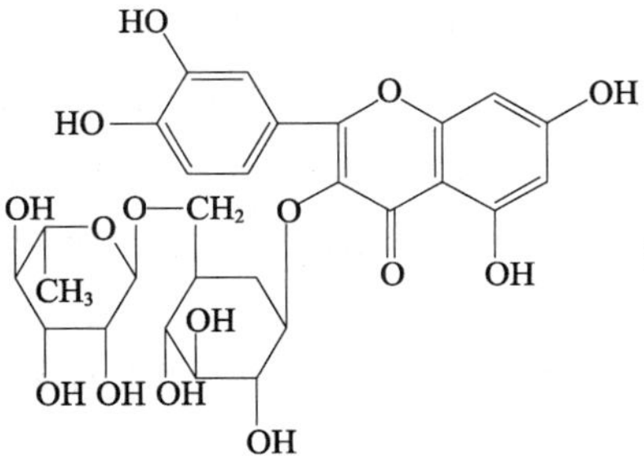

rutin

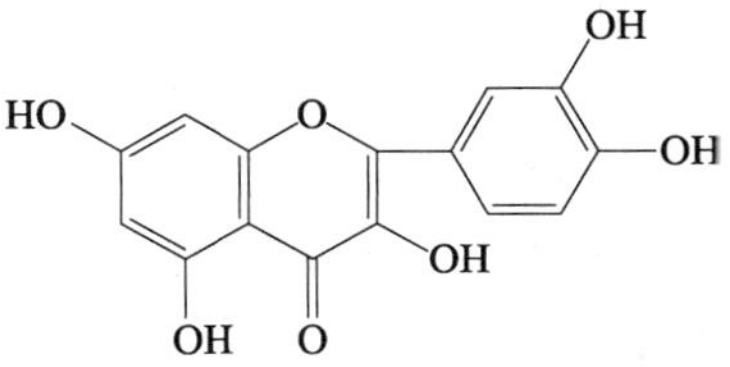

quercetin

3. Physical and chemical properties

(1) Rutin ($C_{27}H_{30}O_{16}$): The molecular weight is 610.51; pale yellow needles (water); the melting point is 176 ~ 178℃, heat to 185 ~ 192℃ turn brown, decomposition point 215℃; $[\alpha]_D^{23}$ + 13.82° (ethanol); UV λ_{Max}^{MeOH} nm: 258, 361; it dissolves in DMSO, pyridine, formyl and aqueous alkali. It's slightly soluble in ethanol, acetone and ethyl acetate, and insoluble in water, chloroform, ether, benzene, petroleum and carbon disulfide.

(2) Quercetin ($C_{15}H_{10}O_7$): The molecular weight is 302.23; yellow crystals (dilute ethanol); anhydride in 95 ~ 97℃; the melting point is 314℃; UV λ_{Max}^{EtOH} nm (logε): 258 (2.75), 375 (2.75); it dissolves in cold ethanol (1:290), easily soluble in boiling ethanol (1:23), soluble in methanol, glacial acetic acid, acetone and ethyl acetate, insoluble in water, chloroform, ether, benzene, petroleum.

4. Actions and indications To cool the blood to stanch bleeding, clear the liver and purge *fire*. Bloody stool, hemorrhoid bleeding, blood dysentery, flooding and spotting, hematemesis, epistaxis, red eyes caused by liver – heat, headache and dizziness.

实验二 山楂叶中黄酮类成分的定性定量分析

【实验目的】

1. 掌握黄酮类成分的性质及其定性定量方法。
2. 掌握聚酰胺薄层色谱法的原理及其在黄酮类成分定性中的应用。
3. 掌握高效液相色谱法的使用。

【实验原理】

1. 聚酰胺薄层色谱法的原理 聚酰胺薄层色谱是一种特殊形式的吸附色谱。常用于黄酮类成分的分析。黄酮类成分中含有酚羟基，而聚酰胺分子中含有酰胺基，二者形成氢键。由于各种黄酮类成分取代基因的性质、多少和位置的不同，与聚酰胺形成氢键的能力有所差异而得到分离。

2. 高效液相色谱法的原理 高效液相色谱法是用高压输液泵将具不同极性的单一溶剂或不同比例的混合溶剂，缓冲液等流动相泵入装有固定相的色谱柱，经进样阀注入供试品，由流动相带入柱内，在柱内各组分被分离后，依次进入检测器，色谱信号由记录仪或积分仪记录。常用的色谱柱填充剂有硅胶和化学键合硅胶，后者以十八烷基键合硅胶最为常用。物质根据其极性大小不同而得到分离。常用的检测器有紫外检测器、二极管阵列检测器、示差折光检测器等。黄酮类化合物由于具有紫外吸收，因此，紫外检测器常用于黄酮类化合物的分析。通常通过比较保留值（通常是保留时间）的方法来鉴定色谱峰。常用的定量方法包括内标法及外标法，外标法最为常用，当用紫外检测器时，其根据物质的峰面积与浓度成正比，计算出样品中待测物质的含量。

【实验器材】

1. 仪器 紫外分光光度计，移液管，容量瓶，锥形瓶，量筒，三用紫外分析仪，水浴锅，超声仪，冷凝管，展开缸，索氏提取器。

2. 试药与试剂 山楂叶药材，芦丁对照品，金丝桃苷对照品，聚酰胺薄层板，乙醇，芦丁，金丝桃苷，石油醚，乙酸乙酯，丙酮，水，三氯甲烷，10%三氯化铝乙醇溶液，氢氧化钠试液，10%硝酸铝溶液，5%亚硝酸钠溶液乙醚。

【实验步骤】

1. 定性分析 取本品粉末2g，加稀乙醇50ml，加热回流1.5小时，放冷，滤过，滤液蒸至无醇味，加水10ml，用石油醚（30 ~ 60℃）洗涤2次，每次20ml，弃去石油醚液，水液加乙酸乙酯振摇提取 2 次，每次 20ml，合并乙酸乙酯液，蒸干，残渣加乙醇 2ml 使溶解，作为供试品溶液。另取芦丁对照品、金丝桃苷对照品，加乙醇分别制成每 1ml 含 0. 1mg 的溶液，作为对照品溶液。照薄层色谱法试验，吸取上述三种溶液各 1 ~2μl，分别点于同一聚酰胺薄膜上，以乙醇 - 丙酮 - 水（7∶5∶6）为展开剂，展开，取出，晾干，喷以三氯化铝试液，热风吹干，置紫外光灯（365nm）下检视。供试品色谱中，在与对照品色谱相应的位置上，显相同颜色的荧光斑点。

2. 定量分析

（1）总黄酮的含量测定

①对照品溶液的制备　精密称取在 120℃ 干燥至恒重的芦丁对照品 25mg，置 50ml 量瓶中，加乙醇适量，超声处理使溶解，放冷，加乙醇至刻度，摇匀。精密量取 20ml，置 50ml 量瓶中，加水至刻度，摇匀，即得（每 1ml 中含无水芦丁 0. 2mg）。

②标准曲线的制备　精密量取对照品溶液 1ml、2ml、3ml、4ml、5ml、6ml，分别置 25ml 量瓶中，各加水至 6ml，加 5% 亚硝酸钠溶液 1ml，摇匀，放置 6 分钟，加 10% 硝酸铝溶液 1ml，摇匀，放置 6 分钟，加氢氧化钠试液 10ml，再加水至刻度，摇匀，放置 15 分钟，以相应试剂为空白，立即照紫外 - 可见分光光度法，在 500nm 的波长处测定吸光度，以吸光度为纵坐标，浓度为横坐标，绘制标准曲线。

③测定法　取本品细粉约 1g，精密称定，置索氏提取器中，加三氯甲烷加热回流提取至提取液无色，弃去三氯甲烷液，药渣挥去三氯甲烷，加甲醇继续提取至无色（约 4 小时），提取液蒸干，残渣加稀乙醇溶解，转移至 50ml 量瓶中，加稀乙醇至刻度，摇匀，作为供试品贮备液。取供试品贮备液，滤过，精密量取续滤液 5ml，置 25ml 量瓶中，加水稀释至刻度，摇匀。精密量取 2ml，置 25ml 量瓶中，照标准曲线制备项下的方法，自“加水至 6ml”起依法测定吸光度，从标准曲线上读出供试品溶液中芦丁的重量，计算，即得。

（2）山楂叶中金丝桃苷的测定

①色谱条件与系统适用性试验　以十八烷基硅烷键合硅胶为填充剂；以乙腈 - 甲醇 - 四氢呋喃 -0. 5% 醋酸溶液（1∶1∶19. 4 ∶78. 6）为流动相；流速：1. 0ml/min；检测波长为 363nm。理论板数按金丝桃苷峰计算应不低于 3000。

②对照品溶液的制备　取金丝桃苷对照品适量，精密称定，加稀乙醇制成每 1ml 含 20μg 的溶液，即得。

③供试品溶液的制备　取“定量分析”总黄酮项下的供试品贮备液，滤过，取续滤液，即得。

④测定法　分别精密吸取对照品溶液与供试品溶液各 10μl，注入液相色谱，测定，即得。

【实验记录】

1. 绘制定性薄层图，记录芦丁、金丝桃苷在本实验的薄层色谱条件下的 R_f 值。

2. 外标一点法计算出药材中金丝桃苷的含量。

【思考题】

1. 芦丁和金丝桃苷的 R_f 值哪个大，为什么？

2. 流动相中为什么要加入四氢呋喃 -0. 5% 醋酸溶液？

【相关资料】

1. 药材来源 本品为蔷薇科植物山里红 *Crataegus pinnatifida* Bge. var. major N. E. Br. 或山楂 *Crataegus pinnatifida* Bge. 的干燥叶。夏、秋二季采收，晾干。

2. 化学成分 目前，人们从山楂叶中分离了很多黄酮类的成分、有机酸类化合物及一些微量元素化合物。黄酮类化合物为山楂叶的主要活性成分。现已分离的主要有：槲皮素、芦丁、金丝桃苷、牡荆素、牡荆素鼠李糖苷、6″－O－乙酰基牡荆素、2″－O－乙酰基牡荆素、牡荆素 2″－O－鼠李糖苷等。2015 版《中国药典》规定，本品按干燥品计算，含总黄酮以无水芦丁（$C_{27}H_{30}O_{16}$）计，不得少于 7.0%（紫外可见分光光度法）。此外，本品按干燥品计算，含金丝桃苷（$C_{21}H_{20}O_{12}$）不得少于 0.050%（高效液相色谱法）。

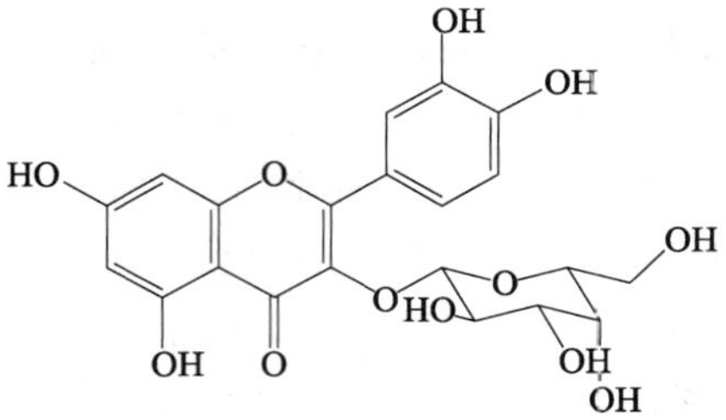

金丝桃苷

3. 理化性质

（1）芦丁：见本章实验一。

（2）金丝桃苷（$C_{21}H_{20}O_{12}$，又名槲皮素－3－*O*－*β*－*D*－吡喃半乳糖苷）：属于黄酮醇苷类化合物，苷元为槲皮素，糖基为吡喃半乳糖，由槲皮素的 3 位 O 原子以 β 糖苷键与糖基相连。分子量为 464.38，淡黄色针状结晶（乙醇）。熔点 227～229℃，旋光度－83°（c＝0.2，吡啶）。易溶于乙醇、甲醇、丙酮和吡啶，通常条件下稳定。UV λ_{Max}^{EtOH}：361（4.38）、258（4.46）、209（4.67）。

4. 功效主治 活血化瘀，理气通脉，化浊降脂。用于气滞血瘀，胸痹心痛，胸闷憋气，心悸健忘，眩晕耳鸣，高脂血症。

Experiment 2 The Qualitative and Quantitative Analysis of Flavonoids in Crataegi Folium

Purpose

1. Comprehend the qualitative analysis and quantitative analysis of flavonoids.
2. Comprehend the principle and operation of Polyamide thin layer chromatography.
3. Comprehend the principle and operation of HPLC through this experiment.

Principle

1. Polyamide thin layer Polyamide is amacromolecule with repeating units linked by amide bonds. Applications of polyamide as the stationary phase in TLC are numerous because any analyte that can undergo H – bonding with the amide are possible. Flavonoids contain many hydroxyl groups which can form H – bonding with the amide. Therefore, polyamide is commonly used as the stationary phase for the separation of flavonoids by TLC. Different flavonoids contain different number of hydroxyl groups or their hydroxyl groups are in the different positions, all of which might result in the different ability in forming H – bond with amide. This difference is responsible for the separation of compounds.

2. High performance liquid chromatography (HPLC) In HPLC, the mobile phase, a solvent or solvent mixture of suitable polarity (or a buffer solution of suitable ion strength) is pumped through injector. While the sample is injected into an injector and carried into the column by the mobile phase, the components are separated on the stationary phase and each component passes through the detector in succession and a chromatogram is thus recorded. The stationary phase and the component part of the mobile phase should be in the accordance with the qualities of test sample. Silica gel and chemically bonded silica gel are commonly used as the packing. For chemically bonded silica gel, octadecylsilane type is the most useful one. The kinds of detector have UV, DAD, SPD and so on. As flavonoids have good absorption under UV light, UV detector is commonly used in the analysis of flavonoids. Retention time (t_R) is used for the identification of compounds. In addition, both internal and external standard methods can be used in the quantification. The peak area is usually directly proportional to the concentration of compound if we use UV detector, thus we can calculate the concentration of the sample.

Conditions

1. Apparatus Ultraviolet detector, three ultraviolet analyzer, Soxhlet's extractor, pipette, volumetric flask, conical flask, measuring cylinder, water bath, ultrasonic wave instrument, developing tank and condenser pipe.

2. Reagents and materials Folium Crataegi, hyperoside CRS, rutin CRS, Polyamide thin layer board, petroleum ether, ethanol, hyperoside, ethyl acetate, chloroform, water, 10% aluminum trichloride in ethanol, acetone, 5% sodium nitrate, sodium hydroxide solution and 10% aluminum nitrate.

Experimental Procedure

1. Qualitative analysis To 2g of the powder, add 50ml of dilute ethanol TS, heat under reflux for 1.5hours, cool, filter, evaporate the filtrate until no ethanol remained, add 10ml of water, wash with two 20ml quantities of petroleum ether (30 ~ 60℃), discard the petroleum ether solutions, extract the water solution with two 20ml quantities of ethyl acetate, combine the ethyl acetate extracts, evaporate to dryness, dissolve the residue in 2ml of ethanol as the test solution. Dissolve rutin CRS and hyperoside CRS in ethanol to prepare two solutions containing 0.1mg of each per ml as the reference solutions. Carry out the method for thin layer chromatography, using polyamide as the coating substance and a mixture of ethanol, acetone and water (7:5:6) as the mobile phase. Apply separately to the film 1 ~ 2μl of each of the above three solutions. After developing and removal of the film, dry in air, spray with aluminum chloride TS, heat under a current of hot air to dryness, and examine under ultraviolet light at 365nm. The fluorescent spots in the chromatogram obtained with the test solution correspond in position and colour to the spots in the chromatogram obtained with the reference solutions.

2. Quantitative analysis

(1) Determination of the content of total flavonoids in Crataegi Folium

①Reference solution Weigh accurately 25mg of rutin CRS (previously dried to constant weight at 120℃), in a 50ml volumetric flask, add a quantity of ethanol, ultrasonicate to dissolve, cool, add ethanol to volume and mix well. Measure accurately 20ml of the solution to a 50ml volumetric flask, add water to volume and mix well to prepare a solution containing 0.2mg of anhydrous rutin per ml as the reference soution.

②Calibration standard Measure accurately 1ml, 2ml, 3ml, 4ml, 5ml and 6ml of the reference solution, respectively, into a 25ml volumetric flask, add water to 6ml, add lml of 5% sodium nitrate, mix well, allow to stand for 6 minutes, add 1ml of 10% aluminum nitrate, mix well and stand for 6 minutes. Add 10ml of sodium hydroxide TS and dilute with water to volume, mix well, stand for 15minutes. Carry out the method for ultraviolet spectrophotometry and colourimetry, using the corresponding solvent as a blank, immediately measure the absorbance at 500nm and plot the standard curve, using absorbance as ordinate and concentration as abscissa.

③Procedure Weigh accurately 1g of the fine powder into a Soxhlet's extractor, add chloroform, and heat under reflux until the extract colorless. Discard the chloroform extract and expel solvent remained in the residue, add methanol, heat under reflux for about 4 hours until the extract colorless, and evaporate the methanol extract to dryness, Dissolve the residue in dilute ethanol TS, transfer to a 50ml volumetric flask, add dilute ethanol TS to volume, mix well as the stock solution. Filter the stock solution, measure accurately 5ml of the successive filtrate to a 25ml volumetric flask, dilute with water to volume and mix well. Measure accurately 2ml of the solution to a 25ml volumetric flask, carry out the procedure as described under the calibration standard beginning at the words "add water to 6ml" to "measure the absorbance at 500nm", read out the weight of rutin in the test solution from the standard curve, and calculate the content.

(2) Determination of the content of hyperoside in Crataegi Folium

①Chromatographic system and system suitability Use octadecylsilane bonded silica gel as the stationary phase and a mixture of acetonitrile, methanol, tetrahydrofuran and 0.5% acetic acid (1:1:19.4:78.6) as the mobile phase. The flow rate: 1.0ml/min. As detector a spectrophotometer set at 363nm. The number of theoretical plates of the column is not less than 3000, calculated with reference to the peak of hyperoside.

②Reference solution Dissolve a quantity of hyperoside CRS, weighed accurately, in dilute ethanol TS to prepare a solution containing 20μg per ml.

③Test solution　Measure the stock solution obtained under the Assay of total flavonoids, filter and use the successive filtrate as the test solution.

④Procedure　Inject accurately 10μl of each of the reference solution and the test solution, respectively, into the column, and calculate the content.

Experimental Records

1. Draw the thin layer chromatogram of identification and calculate R_f value of hyperoside and rutin.

2. Calculate the content of hyperoside in Crataegi Folium.

Questions

1. Compare R_f values of hyperoside and rutin, which is bigger, why?

2. Why do we add terahydrofuran and 0.5% acetic acid in mobile phase?

Background Information

1. Origins　Crataegi Folium is the dried leaf of *Crataegus pinnatifida* Bge. var. major N. E. Br. or *Crataegus pinnatifida* Bge. (Fam. Rosaceae). The drug is collected in summer and autumn, and dried in air.

2. Chemical constituents　Flavonoid, organic acid and trace element were separated from Crataegi Folium. Its principal active component is flavonoids. Various of flavonoids including quercetin, rutin, hyperin, vitexin, rhamnosylvitexin have been separated from Crataegi Folium.

In People's Republic of China Pharmacopoeia (2015 edition), it contains not less than 7.0 percent of flavonoids [calculated as anhydrous rutin ($C_{27}H_{30}O_{16}$)] and 0.050 per cent of hyperoside ($C_{21}H_{20}O_{12}$), calculated with reference to the dried drug.

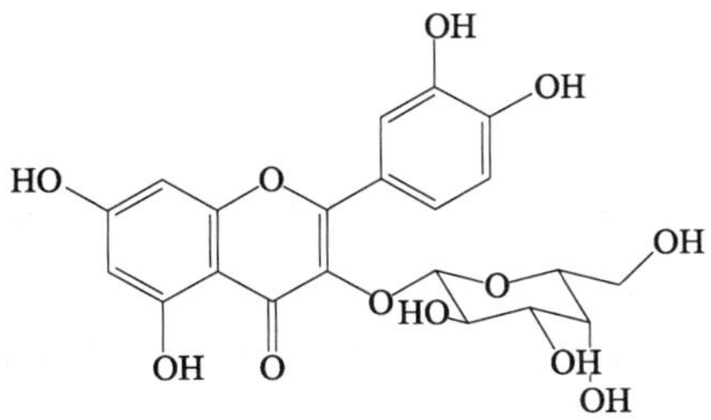

hyperin

3. Physical and chemical properties　Hyperin ($C_{21}H_{20}O_{12}$, quercetin-3-*O*-*β*-*D*-pyran galactose glucoside): The molecular weight is 464.38; pale yellow needles (ethanol); the melting point is 227 ~ 229℃; optical rotation −83° (c = 0.2, pyridine); UV λ_{Max}^{EtOH} nm (logε): 361 (4.38), 258 (4.46), 209 (4.67). It is easily soluble in ethanol, methanol, acetone and pyridine.

4. Actions and indications　To activate blood to resolve stasis. Chest impediment and heart pain, oppression in the chest and labored breathing, palpitation and forgetfulness, dizziness and tinnitus, hyperlipidemia.

实验三　银杏叶中黄酮类成分的定性定量分析

【实验目的】

1. 掌握银杏叶中黄酮类成分的定性定量方法。

2. 掌握高效液相色谱法的使用。

【实验原理】

银杏黄酮主要是以黄酮苷形式存在，经酸水解后生成黄酮醇类化合物，其主要是槲皮素、山柰素、异鼠李素三种成分，本实验用高效液相色谱法测定其含量，再换算成总黄酮醇苷的含量。

【实验器材】

1. 仪器　高效液相色谱仪，紫外检测器，微量进样器，索氏提取器，三用紫外分析仪。

2. 试药与试剂　槲皮素对照品，山柰酚对照品，异鼠李素对照品，银杏叶粉末，硅胶 G 板，乙醇，乙酸乙酯，三氯甲烷，丁酮，甲酸，水，3% 三氯化铝乙醇溶液，甲醇，磷酸，甲醇 - 25% 盐酸溶液（4∶1）。

【实验步骤】

1. 定性分析　取本品粉末 1g，加 40% 乙醇 10ml，加热回流 10 分钟，放冷，滤过，取滤液作为供试品溶液。另取银杏叶对照药材 1g，同法制成对照药材溶液。照薄层色谱法试验，吸取上述两种溶液各 6μl，分别点于同一含 4% 醋酸钠的羧甲基纤维素钠溶液为黏合剂制备的硅胶 G 薄层板上，以乙酸乙酯 - 丁酮 - 甲酸 - 水（5∶3∶1∶1）为展开剂，展开，取出，晾干，喷以 3% 三氯化铝乙醇溶液，热风吹干，置紫外光灯（365nm）下检视。供试品色谱中，在与对照药材色谱相应的位置上，显相同颜色的荧光主斑点。

2. 定量分析

（1）色谱条件与系统适用性试验　以十八烷基硅烷键合硅胶为填充剂；以甲醇 - 0.4% 磷酸溶液（50∶50）为流动相；流速：1.0ml/min；检测波长为 360nm。理论板数按槲皮素峰计算应不低于 2500。

（2）对照品溶液的制备　取槲皮素对照品、山柰素对照品、异鼠李素对照品适量，精密称定，加甲醇分别制成每 1ml 各含槲皮素 30μg、山柰素 30μg、异鼠李素 20μg 的混合溶液，即得。

（3）供试品溶液的制备　取本品中粉约 1g，精密称定，置索氏提取器中，加三氯甲烷回流提取 2 小时，弃去三氯甲烷液，药渣挥干，加甲醇回流提取 4 小时，提取液蒸干，残渣加甲醇 25% 盐酸溶液（4∶1）混合溶液 25ml，加热回流 30 分钟，放冷，转移至 50ml 量瓶中，并加甲醇至刻度，摇匀，即得。

（4）测定法　分别精密吸取对照品溶液与供试品溶液各 10μl，注入液相色谱仪，测定，分别计算槲皮素、山柰素和异鼠李素的含量，按下式换算成总黄酮醇苷的含量。

总黄酮醇苷含量 =（槲皮素含量 + 山柰素含量 + 异鼠李素含量）×2.51

本品按干燥品计算，含总黄酮醇苷不得少于 0.40%。

【实验记录】

1. 绘制定性薄层图，记录银杏叶中主要斑点的 R_f 值及颜色。

2. HPLC 法中，利用外标一点法，计算银杏中总黄酮苷的含量。

【思考题】

1. 换算因子 2.51 的含义是什么?

2. 本实验中为什么使用酸性溶液作为流动相?

【相关资料】

1. 药材来源　本品为银杏科植物银杏 *Ginkgo biloba* L. 的干燥叶。秋季叶尚绿时采收，及时干燥。

2. 化学成分　银杏叶主含黄酮和内酯类成分，黄酮成分主要为双黄酮，如银杏双黄酮、异银杏双黄酮、去甲基银杏双黄酮及芸香苷等，苷元有槲皮素、山柰酚、异鼠李素。内酯类成分有银杏内酯 A、B、C、E 等。

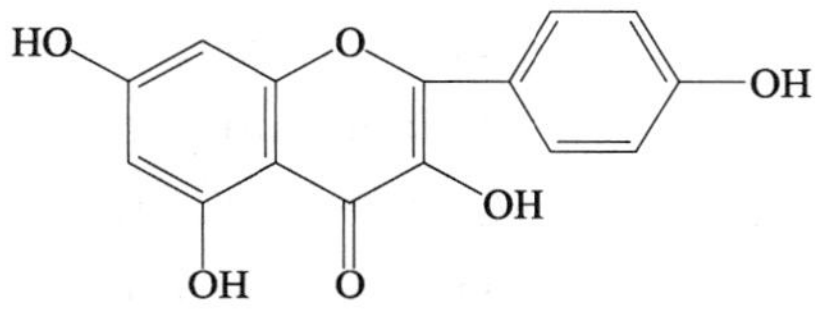

山柰酚

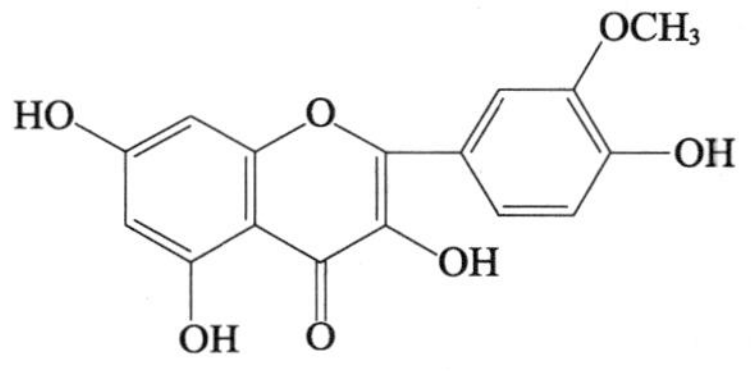

异鼠李素

3. 理化性质

(1) 槲皮素　见本章实验一。

(2) 山柰酚 ($C_{15}H_{10}O_6$)　分子量为 286.23。黄色针状结晶（甲醇），熔点 276 ~ 278℃。微溶于水，溶于热乙醇、乙醚或碱。UV $\lambda_{max}^{CH_3OH}$nm：368 (4.38)，266 (4.35)。二水合物为黄色针状结晶（稀乙醇），在 95 ~ 97℃ 成为无水物，熔点 314℃（分解）。1g 溶于 290ml 无水乙醇、23ml 沸乙醇，溶于冰醋酸，碱性水溶液呈黄色，几乎不溶于水。UV λ_{Max}^{EtOH}nm：258 (2.75)、375 (2.75)。

(3) 异鼠李素 ($C_{16}H_{12}O_7$)　分子量为 316.27。黄色针晶（稀甲醇），熔点 312℃（分解）。UV λ_{max}^{MeOH}nm：257、370。

4. 功效主治　活血化瘀，通络止痛，敛肺平喘，化浊降脂。用于瘀血阻络，胸痹心痛，中风偏瘫，肺虚咳喘，高脂血症。

Experiment 3　The Qualitative and Quantitative Analysis of Flavonoid Constituent in Ginkgo Folium

Purpose

1. Comprehend the principle and operation of HPLC through this experiment.

2. Comprehend the qualitative and quantitative analysis of flavonoid constituents in Ginkgo Folium.

Principle

The chemical substances contained in Ginkgo Folium were reported as flavonol glycosides, which can produce flavonols by acid hydrolysis, such as quercetin, kaempferol and isorhamnetin. In this experiment, we determine the contents of these three substances by HPLC and convert to the content of total amount of flavonol glycosides.

Conditions

1. Apparatus HPLC instrument, microsyringe, ultraviolet analyzer and Soxhlet's extractor.

2. Reagents and materials Crude drug of Ginkgo Folium, quercetin, kaempferol and isorhamnetin CRS, silica gel G, ethanol, ethyl acetate, chloroform, butanone, methanoic acid, phosphoric acid, water, 3% Aluminum trichloride in ethanol, methanol and methanol – 25% hydrochloric acid (4∶1).

Experimental Procedure

1. Qualitative analysis To 1g of the powder add 10ml of methanol, heat under reflux for 10minutes, cool, filter, and use the filtrate as the test solution. Prepare a solution with 1g of Ginkgo Folium reference drug in the same manner as the reference drug solution. Carry out the method for thin layer chromatography, using silica gel G mixed with 4% sodium acetate as the coating substance and a mixture of ethyl acetate, butanone, formic acid and water (5∶3∶1∶1) as the mobile phase. Apply separately to the plate 6μl of each of the above two solutions. After developing and removal of the plate, dry in air, spray with a 3% solution of aluminum chloride in ethanol, heat to dry, and examine under ultraviolet light at 365nm. The main fluorescent spots in the chromatogram obtained with the test solution correspond in position and color to the spots in the chromatogram obtained with the reference drug solution.

2. Quantitative Analysis

(1) Chromatographic system and system suitability Use octadecylsilane bonded silica gel as the stationary phase and methanol – 0.4% phosphoric acid solution (50∶50) as the mobile phase. The flow rate: 1.0ml/min. As detector a spectrophotometer set at 360nm. The number of theoretical plates of the column is not less than 2500, calculated with reference to the peak of quercetin.

(2) Reference solution Weigh accurately a quantity of quercetin CRS, kaempferol CRS and isorhamnetin CRS, previously dried overnight over phosphorous pentoxide, dissolve in methanol to prepare a mixture containing 30μg of each of quercetin and kaempferol and 20μg of isorhamnetin per ml as the reference solution.

(3) Test solution Weigh accurately 1g of the powder into a Soxhlet's extractor, add chloroform and heat under reflux for 2 hours. Discard the chloroform solution, evaporate the residue to dryness, add methanol, heat under reflux for 4 hours, and evaporate the extract to dryness. Dissolve the residue in 25ml of a mixture of methanol and 25% hydrochloric acid (4:1), heat under reflux for 30 minutes, cool, transfer to a 50ml volumetric flask, add methanol to volume, and mix well. Filter trough a membrane (particle size 0.45μm), and use the successive filtrate as the test solution.

(4) Procedure　Inject accurately 10μl of each of the reference solution and the test solution, into the column, and calculate the contents of quercetin, kaempferol and isorhamnetin, respectively. Calculate the content of the total amount of flavonol glycosides using the following equation.

The content of total amount of flavonol glycosides = (the content of quercetin + the content of kaempferol + the content of isorhamnetin) ×2.51.

Experimental Records

1. Draw the thin layer chromatogram and calculate R_f value of the main spots in Ginkgo Folium.

2. Calculate the content of total flavonol glycosides in Ginkgo Folium.

Questions

1. What is the meaning of the conversion factor 2.51?

2. Why do we use acid mobile phase in this experiment?

Background Information

1. Origins　Ginkgo Folium is the dried leaf of *Ginkgo biloba* L. (Fam. Ginkgoaceae). The drug is collected in autumn when leaf green, and dried immediately.

2. Chemical constituents　Ginkgo Folium mainly contains flavonoid (mainly biflavone) and lactones. Many flavonoids such as ginkgetin, isoginkgetin, demethylation - ginkgetin and rutin have been isolated. Their aglycones are quercetin, kaempferol, isorhamnetin. In addition, many lactones including ginkgolide A, B, C, E and so on have been also isolated.

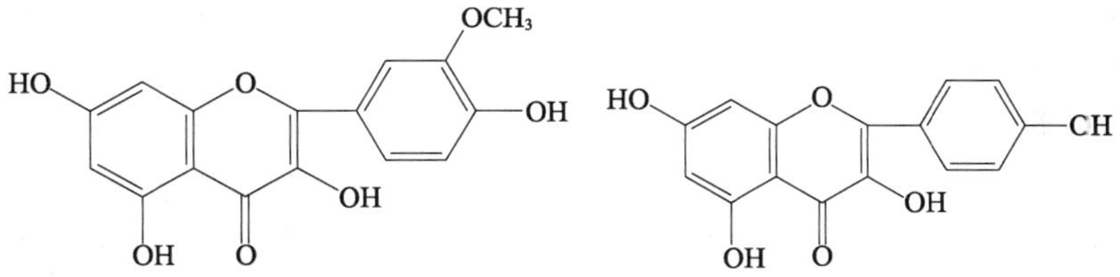

isorhamnetin　　kaempferol

3. Physical and chemical properties

(1) Quercetin　See Experiment 1 of this chapter.

(2) Kaempferol ($C_{15}H_{10}O_6$)　The molecular weight is 286.23; yellow needles (methanol); the melting point is 276 ~ 278℃; UV λ_{Max}^{MeOH} nm (logε): 368 (4.38), 266 (4.35). It's slightly soluble in water, dissolves in boiling ethanol, ethyl acetate and alkali.

(3) Isorhamnetin ($C_{16}H_{12}O_7$)　The molecular weight is 316.27; yellow needles (dilute methanol); the melting point is 312℃; UV λ_{max}^{MeOH}nm: 257, 370.

4. Actions and indications　To activate blood to resolve stasis, unblock the collaterals and relieve pain, constrain the lung to relieve panting, resolve turbidity and lower lipid. Obstruction of collaterals by blood stasis, chest impediment and heart pain, hemiplegia caused by windstroke, cough and panting caused by lung deficiency, hyperlipidemia.

实验四　蛇胆陈皮片中黄酮类成分的定性定量分析

【实验目的】

1. 掌握薄层色谱法在中成药定性中的应用。

2. 掌握高效液相色谱法在中成药定量中的应用。

3. 熟悉中成药的定性定量方法。

【实验原理】

蛇胆陈皮片主要有蛇胆汁和陈皮组成，其中蛇胆汁 26g 和陈皮 156g。由于陈皮为君药，故该方的定性定量分析主要以陈皮为主。陈皮中主要含挥发油、黄酮等成分，其中橙皮苷为其主要的黄酮类成分。2015 版《中国药典》规定，本品每片含陈皮以橙皮苷（$C_{28}H_{34}O_{15}$）计，素片不得少于 5. 0mg，薄膜片不得少于 10. 0mg。

【实验器材】

1. 仪器　高效液相色谱仪，索氏提取器，三用紫外分析仪，超声仪，水浴锅。

2. 试药与试剂　橙皮苷对照品，蛇胆陈皮片，硅胶 G 板，乙酸乙酯，三氯甲烷，水，10% 三氯化铝乙醇溶液，甲醇，磷酸，乙腈。

【实验步骤】

1. 定性分析　取本品适量，研细，取约 0. 1g，加甲醇 10ml，超声处理 20 分钟，滤过，滤液作为供试品溶液。另取橙皮苷对照品，加甲醇制成饱和溶液，作为对照品溶液。照薄层色谱法试验，吸取上述两种溶液各 5μl，分别点于同一硅胶 G 薄层板上，以乙酸乙酯－甲醇－水（100∶17∶13）作为展开剂，展开，取出，晾干，喷以 10% 三氯化铝乙醇溶液，置紫外灯（365nm）下检视。供试品色谱中，在与对照品色谱相应的位置上，显相同颜色的荧光斑点。

2. 定量分析

（1）色谱条件与系统适用性试验　以十八烷基硅烷键合硅胶为填充剂；以乙腈－0. 1% 磷酸溶液（22∶78）为流动相；流速：1. 0ml/min；检测波长为 284nm。理论板数按橙皮苷峰计算应不低于 3000。

（2）供试品溶液的制备　取本品，研细，取约 0. 1g，精密称定，精密加入甲醇 50ml，称定重量，加热回流 30 分钟，放冷，称定重量，用甲醇补足减失的重量，摇匀，滤过，取续滤液，即得。

（3）测定法　分别精密吸取对照品溶液与供试品溶液各 5μl，注入液相色谱仪，测定，即得。

【实验记录】

1. 绘制定性薄层图，记录该色谱条件下橙皮苷的 R_f 值及颜色。

2. HPLC 法中，利用外标一点法，计算该中成药中橙皮苷的含量。

【思考题】

请设计一个实验方案对该制剂中的蛇胆汁进行定性定量分析。

【相关资料】

1. 处方、制法及药材来源　本品为棕色的片；气微香，味甘、辛、微苦。口服，常用量，一次2～4片。由蛇胆汁26g和陈皮156g组成。以上二味，陈皮粉碎成细粉，过筛，与蛇胆汁混匀，干燥，研成细粉，加辅料适量，制成颗粒，干燥，压制成片，即得。

其中陈皮为芸香科植物橘 *Citrus reticulate* Blanco 及其栽培变种的干燥成熟果皮。药材分为“陈皮”和“广陈皮”。采摘成熟果实，剥取果皮，晒干或低温干燥。

2. 化学成分 陈皮主含挥发油、黄酮类、有机胺类及微量元素等成分。陈皮挥发油含量约为1.5%～2.0%，广陈皮挥发油含量约为1.2%～3.2%，包括α－侧柏烯、α－蒎烯、桧烯、β－蒎烯等化合物。陈皮中的黄酮类化合物主要以橙皮苷、新橙皮苷、陈皮素、柚皮苷等为主。

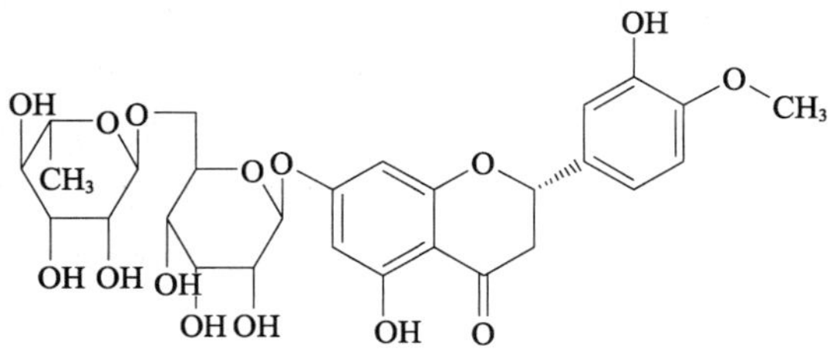

橙皮苷

3. 理化性质 橙皮苷（$C_{28}H_{34}O_{15}$）：分子量为610.56，淡黄色结晶性粉末（甲醇）。熔点：250～255℃。易溶于吡啶、氢氧化钠溶液，溶于二甲基甲酰胺，微溶于甲醇和热冰醋酸，极微溶于乙醚、丙酮、三氯甲烷和苯。该品1g溶于50L水。无臭、无味。

4. 功能主治 顺气除痰，祛风健胃。用于风痰咳嗽，气逆反胃。

（杨杰）

Experiment 4 The Qualitative and Quantitative Analysis of Flavonoid Constituents in Shedan Chenpi Tablets

Purpose

1. Comprehend the application of thin layer chromatography in qualitative analysis of traditional Chinese medicine preparation.

2. Comprehend the application of high performance liquid chromatogram in quantitative analysis of traditional Chinese medicine preparation.

3. Understand the qualitative and quantitative analysis of traditional Chinese medicine preparation.

Principle

Shedan Chenpi Tablets is composed of Pericarpium citri reticulatae (156g) and Fel serpentis (26g). Pericarpium citri reticulatae is the main material in this preparation. The main components in Pericarpium citri reticulatae are essential oils and flavonoids. Hesperidin is one of flavonoids in Pericarpium citri reticulatae.

Conditions

1. Apparatus HPLC instrument, ultraviolet analyzer, Soxhlet's extractor, water bath and ultrasonic cleaner.

2. Reagents and materials Shedan chenpi tablets, naringenin CRS, silica gel G, ethyl acetate, chloroform, methanol, phosphoric acid, water, 3% Aluminum trichloride in ethanol and acetonitrile.

Experimental Procedure

1. Qualitative analysis Grind a quantity of coated tablets to fine powder, weigh 0. 1g and add 10ml of methanol, ultrasonicate for 20 minutes, filter and use the filtrate as the test solution. Dissolve naringenin CRS in methanol to prepare a saturated solution as the reference solution. Carry out the method for thin layer chromatography, using silica gel G as the coating substance and a mixture of ethyl acetate, methanol and water (100∶17∶13) as the mobile phase. Apply separately 5μl of the above two solutions to the plate. After developing and removal of the plate, dry in air, spray with 10% aluminum chloride in ethanol, examine under ultraviolet light at 365nm. The fluorescent spots in the chromatogram obtained with the test solution correspond in position and color to the spots in the chromatogram obtained with the reference solution.

2. Quantitative analysis

(1) Chromatographic system and system suitability Use octadecylsilane bonded silica gel as the stationary phase and a mixture of acetonitrile and 0. 1% phosphoric acid (22∶78) as the mobile phase. The flow rate: 1. 0ml/min. As detector a spectrophotometer set at 284nm. The number of theoretical plates of the column is not less than 3000, calculated with reference to the peak of naringenin.

(2) Reference solution Weigh accurately a quantity of naringenin CRS, dissolve in methanol to prepare a mixture containing 40μg per ml as the reference solution.

(3) Test solution Weigh accurately 0. 1g of the powder, add accurately 50ml of methanol and weigh. Heat under reflux for 30 minutes, cool and weigh again, replenish the loss of weight with methanol, mix well, filter and use the successive filtrate as the test solution.

(4) Procedure Inject accurately 5μl of each of the above reference solution and the test solution into the column, determine and calculate the content of naringenin in this preparation.

Experimental Records

1. Draw the thin layer chromatogram and calculate R_f value of naringenin.

2. Calculate the content of naringenin in this preparation.

Questions

Design an experiment to deal with the qualitative analysis and quantitative analysis of Serpentis Felin in this preparation.

Background Information

1. Origins Citri Reticulatae Pericarpium is dried ripe peel of *Citrus reticulata* Blanco and its cultivated varieties of Rutaceae family. Medicine is divided into "chenpi" and "guangchenpi" . Pick ripe fruit and strip the skin, dry or dry at low temperature.

2. Chemical constituents Citri Reticulatae Pericarpium mainly contains essential oil, flavonoid, organic amine and trace element. The content of essential oil in Citri Reticulatae Pericarpium is up to 1.5% ~2.0% and 1.2% ~3.2% in guangchenpi. The compounds in essential oil are including α - pinene, α - thujene, β - pinene and so on. Many flavonoids including hesperidin, neohesperidin, neobiletin and naringin have also been isolated.

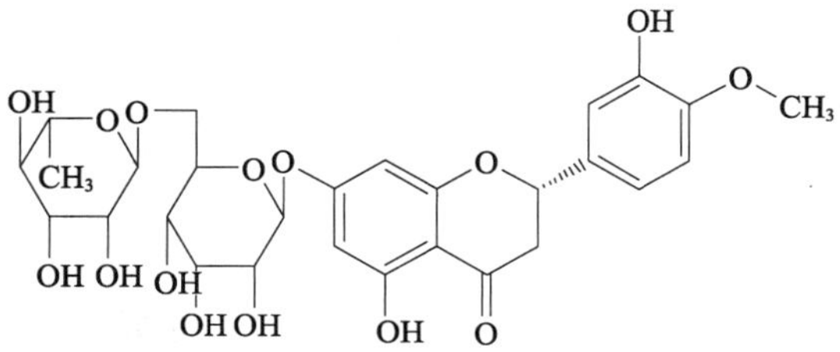

hesperidin

3. Physical and chemical properties Hesperidin ($C_{28}H_{34}O_{15}$): The molecular weight is 610.56; pale yellow crystal powder (methanol); the melting point is 250 ~ 255℃; it's easily soluble in pyridine, sodium hydroxide solution, soluble in dimethylformamide, slightly soluble in methanol and boiling glacial acetic acid. 1g of this compound can dissolve in 50L water. It is odourless and tasteless.

4. Actions and indications To regulate *qi* and resolve phlegm. Cough, vomiting and hiccup caused by phlegm turbidity obstructing the lung, stomach *qi* rising.

(Jie Yang)

第三章
醌类成分的分析

实验一　大黄中蒽醌类化合物的定性定量分析

【实验目的】

1. 掌握蒽醌类成分的性质及其定性定量方法。
2. 掌握薄层色谱法的操作技术及其在蒽醌类成分定性中的应用。
3. 掌握紫外可见分光光度法在蒽醌类化合物含量测定中的应用。

【实验原理】

1. 薄层色谱法　蒽醌类化合物的吸附剂多用硅胶。展开剂多为混合溶剂，因蒽醌类化合物多含酚羟基，在展开剂中常加入酸，改善其拖尾。由于蒽醌类化合物大多具有紫外吸收且能和碱液反应而显色。因此，显色剂多用碱液显色，或置于紫外灯下观察。

2. 比色法　该方法是依据蒽醌类成分与碱液或醋酸镁试液生成红色，于 500 ~ 550nm 处有最大吸收，进行比色法测定。蒽酮、蒽酚、二蒽酮类必须被氧化成蒽醌后才会呈阳性反应。蒽醌类化合物具有多种结构，根据其是否接糖分为苷元（游离蒽醌）及苷类（结合蒽醌），或根据其氧化程度分为氧化型蒽醌及还原型蒽醌（蒽酚、蒽酮、二蒽酮），不同类型的蒽醌在一定的条件下能发生相互转化，如下图所示：

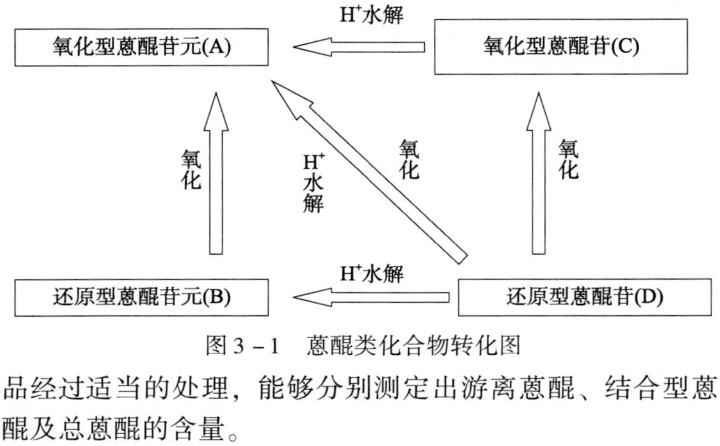

图 3－1　蒽醌类化合物转化图

因此，样品经过适当的处理，能够分别测定出游离蒽醌、结合型蒽醌或氧化型蒽醌、还原型蒽醌及总蒽醌的含量。

【实验器材】

1. 仪器　高效液相色谱仪、紫外可见分光光度计、三用紫外仪、移液管、容量瓶、锥形瓶、量筒、展开缸。

2. 试药与试剂　大黄药材，芦荟大黄素对照品，大黄酸对照品，大黄素对照品，大黄酚对照品，大黄素甲醚对照品，1，8－二羟基蒽醌，硅胶H薄层板，甲醇，水，乙醚，$NaHCO_3$，10% $FeCl_3$溶液，浓盐酸，三氯甲烷，0.5%醋酸镁甲醇溶液。

【实验步骤】

1. 定性分析

（1）取本品粉末少量，进行微量升华，可见菱状针晶或羽状结晶。

（2）取本品粉末0.1g，加甲醇20ml，浸泡1小时，滤过，取滤液5ml，蒸干，残渣加水10ml使溶解，再加盐酸1ml，加热回流30分钟，立即冷却，用乙醚分2次振摇提取，每次20ml，合并乙醚液，蒸干，残渣加三氯甲烷1ml使溶解，作为供试品溶液。另取大黄对照药材0.1g，同法制成对照药材溶液。再取大黄酸对照品，加甲醇制成每1ml含1mg的溶液，作为对照品溶液。照薄层色谱法试验，吸取上述三种溶液各4μl，分别点于同一以羧甲基纤维素钠为黏合剂的硅胶H薄层板上，以石油醚（30～60℃）－甲酸乙酯－甲酸（15∶5∶1）的上层溶液为展开剂，展开，取出，晾干，置紫外光灯（365nm）下检视。供试品色谱中，在与对照药材色谱相应的位置上，显相同的五个橙黄色荧光主斑点；在与对照品色谱相应的位置上，显相同的橙黄色荧光斑点，置氨蒸气中熏后，斑点变为红色。

2. 定量分析

（1）大黄中总蒽醌的含量测定

①对照品溶液及标准曲线　精密称取1，8－二羟基蒽醌2.5mg于25ml容量瓶中，加三氯甲烷溶解并加至刻度，精密吸取对照品溶液0.5、1、2、3、4ml，分别置于25ml容量瓶中，蒸去三氯甲烷，加0.5% 醋酸镁甲醇溶液至刻度，摇匀。以甲醇为空白，在515nm处测定，以吸收度为纵坐标，浓度（μg/ml）为横坐标，绘图。

②供试品溶液的制备　精密称取药材粉末0.1g，置100ml烧瓶中，精密加入水25ml，称定重量。置水浴中回流加热15分钟，放冷，称定重量，用水补足至原重量，加碳酸氢钠50mg，摇匀，静置后用干燥滤纸滤过，弃去初滤液，精密吸取续滤液10ml，置100ml具塞烧瓶中，加10% $FeCl_3$溶液20ml，水浴回流20分钟，加HCl 1ml，继续回流30分钟，放冷，加入三氯甲烷25ml，盖好瓶盖，用力振摇，转移至125ml分液漏斗中，使分层，分取三氯甲烷层，再用25ml 三氯甲烷（洗涤烧瓶后）萃取一次，分取三氯甲烷层与上次合并，并用水洗涤二次，每次用水15ml，将三氯甲烷层用干燥滤纸滤过于100ml容量瓶中，用三氯甲烷洗涤滤纸，洗液合并于容量瓶中，用三氯甲烷稀释至刻度，摇匀。精密吸取10ml三氯甲烷提取液，置25ml具塞烧瓶中，蒸去三氯甲烷，放冷，精密加入0.5% 醋酸镁甲醇溶液10ml，摇匀。

③测定法　以甲醇为空白，在515nm处测定吸收值，由标准曲线计算含量。

（2）HPLC法测定大黄中蒽醌类化合物的含量

①色谱条件与系统适用性试验　以十八烷基硅烷键合硅胶为填充剂；以甲醇－0.1%磷酸溶液（85∶15）为流动相；流速：1.0ml/min；检测波长为254nm。理论板数

按大黄素峰计算应不低于3000。

②对照品溶液的制备　精密称取芦荟大黄素对照品、大黄酸对照品、大黄素对照品、大黄酚对照品、大黄素甲醚对照品适量，加甲醇分别制成每1ml含芦荟大黄素、大黄酸、大黄素、大黄酚各80μg，大黄素甲醚40μg的溶液；分别精密量取上述对照品溶液各2ml，混匀，即得（每1ml中含芦荟大黄素、大黄酸、大黄素、大黄酚各16μg，含大黄素甲醚8μg）。

③供试品溶液的制备　取本品粉末（过四号筛）约0.15g，精密称定，置具塞锥形瓶中，精密加入甲醇25ml，称定重量，加热回流1小时，放冷，再称定重量，用甲醇补足减失的重量，摇匀，滤过。精密量取续滤液5ml，置烧瓶中，挥去溶剂，加8%盐酸溶液10ml，超声处理2分钟，再加三氯甲烷10ml，加热回流1小时，放冷，置分液漏斗中，用少量三氯甲烷洗涤容器，并入分液漏斗中，分取三氯甲烷层，酸液再用三氯甲烷提取3次，每次10ml，合并三氯甲烷液，减压回收溶剂至干，残渣加甲醇使溶解，转移至10ml量瓶中，加甲醇至刻度，摇匀，滤过，取续滤液，即得。

④测定法　分别精密吸取对照品溶液与供试品溶液各10μl，注入液相色谱仪，测定，即得。

【实验记录】

1. 绘制定性薄层图，记录大黄药材中主要斑点的R_f值

2. 比色法中，绘标准曲线图，并计算大黄中结合蒽醌和游离大黄酸的总含量。

【思考题】

1. 加水提取的是何类成分，加入10% $FeCl_3$的目的是什么？

2. 加入浓盐酸的目的是什么？

3. 用比色法测定蒽醌类成分应注意什么？

【相关资料】

1. 药材来源　大黄为蓼科植物掌叶大黄 *Rheum palmatum* L.、唐古特大黄 *Rheum tanguticum* Maxim et Regel 或药用大黄 *Rheum offcihale* Baill 的干燥根和根茎。秋末茎叶枯萎或次春发芽前采挖，除去细根，刮去外皮，切瓣或段，绳穿成串干燥或直接干燥。

2. 化学成分　大黄主含蒽醌类化合物，包括游离及结合状态的大黄酚、大黄酸、芦荟大黄素、大黄素、大黄素甲醚及番泻苷A、B、C、D。2015版《中国药典》规定，本品按干燥品计算（高效液相色谱法），含芦荟大黄素（$C_{15}H_{10}O_5$）、大黄酸（$C_{15}H_8O_6$）、大黄素（$C_{15}H_{10}O_5$）、大黄酚（$C_{15}H_{10}O_4$）和大黄素甲醚（$C_{16}H_{12}O_5$）的总量不得少于1.5%。

3. 理化性质

（1）大黄酸（$C_{15}H_8O_6$）：分子量为284.21。黄色针状结晶（三氯甲烷），熔点321～322℃。几乎不溶于水，溶于碱液，略溶于乙醇、苯、三氯甲烷、乙醚和石油醚。UV λ_{Max}^{MeOH}nm：229、258、435。

（2）大黄素甲醚（$C_{16}H_{12}O_5$）：分子量为284.26。砖红色单斜针状结晶（苯），熔点203～207℃。不溶于甲醇、乙醇、乙醚和丙酮，溶于碱液、苯、三氯甲烷、甲苯。UV λ_{Max}^{EtOH}nm：266、255、267、288、440。

4. 功效主治　泻下攻积，清热泻火，凉血解毒，逐瘀通经，利湿退黄。用于实热

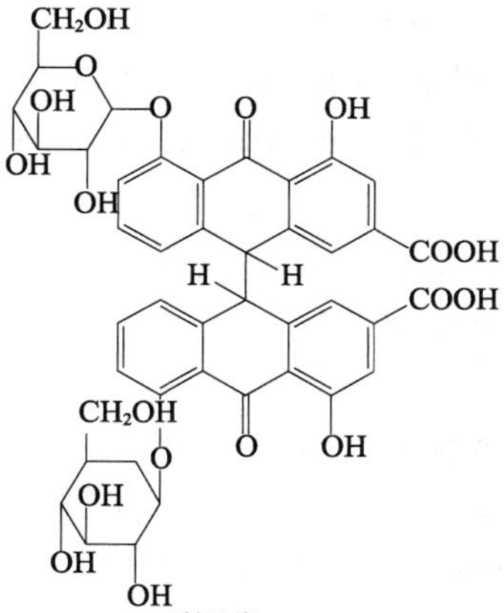

番泻苷

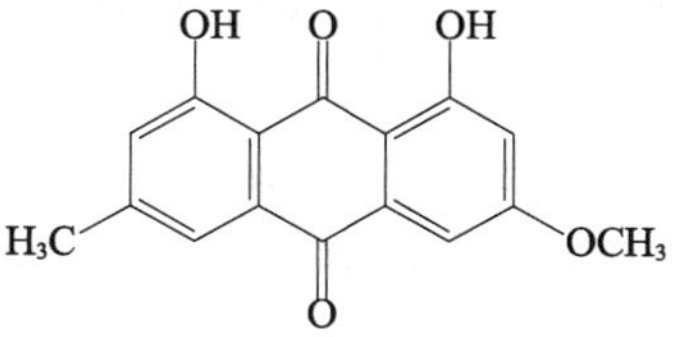

大黄素甲醚

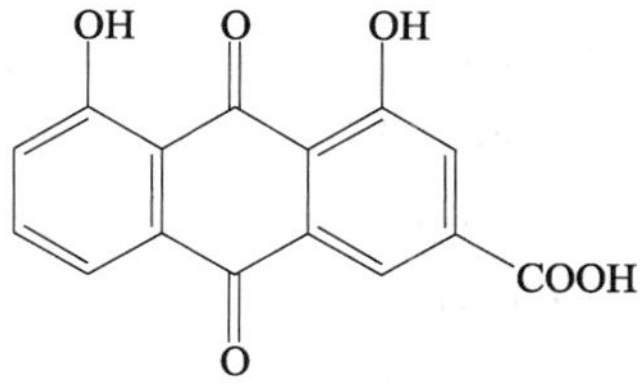

大黄酸

积滞便秘，血热吐衄，目赤咽肿，痈肿疔疮，肠痈腹痛，瘀血经闭，产后瘀阻，跌打损伤，湿热痢疾，黄疸尿赤，淋证，水肿；外治烧烫伤。酒大黄善清上焦血分热毒。用于目赤咽肿，齿龈肿痛。熟大黄泻下力缓，泻火解毒。用于火毒疮疡。大黄炭凉血化瘀止血。用于血热有瘀出血症。

Experiment 1　The Qualitative and Quantitative Analysis of Anthraquinones in Rhei Radix et Rhizoma

Purpose

1. Comprehend the properties of anthraquinones and its qualitative and quantitative methods.

2. Comprehend operation of thin layer chromatography and its application in the qualitative analysis of anthraquinones.

3. Comprehend the application of ultraviolet visible spectrophotometry in the determination of anthraquinone compounds.

Principle

1. Thin layer chromatography　Silica gel is commonly used as the stationary phase for anthraquinone. A solvent mixture is often used as mobile phase. Since anthraquinone always contains hydroxyl groups, the spots tailing might occur in TLC. A solution to remove this tailing is to add acidic solution into the mobile phase. As anthraquinone have good absorption under UV light, the spots of compounds can be seen by illuminating the plate with short-wave UV. A number of chemical stains can be used such as the solution of NaOH or ammonia.

2. Colorimetry　Anthraquinones could react with magnesium acetate solution to generate colored substance, which has a maximum absorption at 500 ~ 550nm. Thus, the content of anthraquinones could be determined by colorimetric method. However, this reaction happens only when anthrone, anthranol, dianthrone are oxidized to anthraquinone. Anthraquinone has a variety of structures. We can classify them into aglycone (free anthraquinone) and glycosides (combined anthraquinone), or into oxidized and reduced anthraquinone according to their degree of oxidation. Different types of anthraquinone can changed into each other under certain conditions.

Thus, these changes could be used to determine the contents of free anthraquinone, combined anthraquinone, oxidized and reduced anthraquinone respectively.

Conditions

1. Apparatus HPLC instrument, ultraviolet visible spectrophotometer, ultraviolet analyzer, pipette, volumetric flask, conical flask, graduated cylinder and expansion cylinder.

2. Reagents and materials Rhei Radix et Rhizoma, aloeemodin CRS, rhein CRS, emodin CRS, chrysophanol CRS, physcion CRS, 1, 8 – dihydroxy – anthraquinone CRS; Silica gel H thin layer plate, methanol, water, ethyl ether, $NaHCO_3$, 10% $FeCl_3$, concentrated hydrochloric acid, chloroform and 0.5% magnesium acetate in methanol.

Experimental Procedure

1. Qualitative analysis

(1) Sublime a small quantity of the powder, rhombic needles or feathery crystal should be visible.

(2) Macerate 0.1g of the powder in 20ml of methanol for 1 hour, and filter. Evaporate 5ml of the filtrate to dryness, dissolve the residue in 10ml of water, add 1ml of hydrochloric acid, heat under reflux on a water bath for 30 minutes and cool immediately. Extract by shaking with two 20ml quantuties of ether, combine the ether extracts, evaporate to dryness and dissolve the residue in 1ml of chloroform as the test solution. Prepare a solution of Rhei Radix et Rhizoma reference drug in the same manner as the reference solution. Dissolve a quantity of rhein CRS in methanol to produce a solution containing 1mg per ml as the reference solution. Carry out the method for thin layer chromatography, using silica gel H mixed with sodium carboxymethylcellulose as the coating substance and upper layer of a mixture of petroleum ether (30 ~ 60℃), ethyl formate and formic acid (15 : 5 : 1) as the mobile phase. Apply separately 4μl of each of the above three solutions to the plate. After developing and removal of the plate, dry in air, and examine under ultraviolet light at 365nm. The five orange fluorescent spots in the chromatogram obtained with the test solution corresponds in position and color to the spots in the chromatogram obtained with the reference drug solution; the orange fluorescent spot in the chromatogram obtained with the test solution correspond in position and color to the spots in the chromatogram obtained with the reference drug solution. The spot becomes red on exposure to ammonia vapour.

2. Quantitative analysis

(1) Determination of total anthraquinones in Rhei Radix et Rhizoma

①Reference solution Weigh accurately 2.5ml of 1, 8 – dihydroxy – anthraquinone to a 25ml volumetric flask, dissolve in chloroform, and dilute to the volume.

②Standard curve Tansfer accurately 0.5ml, 1ml, 2ml, 3ml, 4ml of the reference solution to a 25ml volumetric flask, respectively, evaporate the chloroform, dilute with 0.5% magnesium acetate in methanol to volume, and mix well. Use methanol as the blank, measure the absorbance as ordinate and the concentration (μg/ml) as abscissa.

③Test solution　Weigh accurately 0.1g of the powder to a 100ml conical flask, accurately add 25ml of water and weigh, heat under reflux on a water bath for 15 minutes, allow to cool, weigh again, replenish the loss of the solvent with water, add 50mg of sodium bicarbonate, mix well, and allow to stand, filter through a piece of dry filter paper, discard the initial filtrate, transfer accurately 10ml of the successive filtrate to a 100ml stopper conical flask, add 20ml 10% ferric chloride solution, heat under reflux on a water bath for 20 minutes, add 1ml hydrochloric acid, continue to heat under reflux on a water bath for 30 minutes, allow to cool, add 25ml of chloroform, tightly stopper and shake vigorously, transfer to a 125ml separating funnel, allow to stand, separate the chloroform layer, extract with 25ml of chloroform (wash the flask with it first) again, separate the chloroform layer. Wash the combined chloroform extracts with two 15ml quantities of water. Filter the chloroform extract through a piece of dry filter paper to a 100ml volumetric flask, wash the filter paper with chloroform to the same flask, dilute with chloroform to volume, and mix well. Transfer accurately 10ml of the chloroform solution to a 25ml stopper conical flask, evaporate the chloroform, cool and add accurately 10ml of 0.5% solution of magnesium acetate in methanol, and mix well. Using methanol as the blank, measure the absorbance at 515nm. Calculate the content by the standard curve.

(2) Determination of anthraquinone compounds in Rhei Radix et Rhizoma by HPLC

①Chromatographic system and system suitability　Use octadecylsilane bonded silica gel as the stationary phase and a mixture of methanol and 0.1% phosphoric acid (85∶15) as the mobile phase. The flow rate: 1.0ml/min. As detector a spectrophotometer set at 254nm. The number of theoretical plates of the column is not less than 3000, calculated with the reference to the peak of emodin.

②Reference solution　Weigh accurately a quantity of aloeemodin CRS, rhein CRS, emodin CRS, chrysophanol CRS and physcion CRS, respectively, dissolve in methanol to produce five solutions containing 80μg of each of aloeemodin, rhein, emodin, chrysophanol per ml and 40μg of physcion per ml. Measure accurately 2ml of each above solution to produce a mixture containing 16μg of aloeemodin, rhein, emodin, chrysophanol and 8μg of physcion per ml as the reference solution.

③Test solution　Weigh accurately 0.15g of the powder (through No.4 sieve) to a stopper conical flask, accurately add 25ml of methanol and weigh. Heat under reflux on a water bath for one hour, cool, weigh again, replenish the loss of weight with methanol, mix well and filter. Measure accurately 5ml of successive filtrate in a flask, expel the solvent, add 10ml of 8% solution of hydrochloric acid, ultrasonicate for 2 minutes, add 10ml of chloroform, Heat under reflux for 1 hour, cool, transfer to a separating funnel. Separate the chloroform layer, extract the acid solution again with three 10-ml quantities of chloroform, combine the chloroform extracts and recover the chloroform in a vacuum to dryness. Dissolve the residue in methanol to volume and mix well as the test solution.

④Procedure Accurately inject 10μl of each of the reference solution and the test solution, respectively, into the column, and calculated the content.

Experimental Records

1. Draw the TLC chromatogram and record the R_f values of main compounds.

2. Plot the standard curve of the reference solution and calculate the total content of anthraquinone in the Rhei Radix et Rhizoma.

Questions

1. What kind of components are extracted by water? What's the purpose of adding 10% $FeCl_3$?

2. What's the purpose of adding concentrated hydrochloric acid?

3. Which procedure should we pay more attention to in determining anthraquinone using colorimetric method?

Background Information

1. Origins Rhei Radix et Rhizoma is the dried root and rhizome of *Rheum palmatum* L., *Rheum tanguticum* Maxinm et Regel or *Rheum officinale* Baill (Fam. Polygonaceae). The drug is collected in late autumn when stem and leaves are withered or in next spring just before budding, removed from rootlet and the outer bark. Cut into segment or section, either stringed together to be dried, or dried directly.

2. Chemical constituents Rhei Radix et Rhizoma mainly contains anthraquinone compounds, including Chrysophanol, rhein, aloeemodin, emodin, physcion, sennoside A, B, C, D and so on. In People's Republic of China Pharmacopoeia (2015 edition), it should contain not less than 1.5 percent of the total amount of aloe-emodin ($C_{15}H_{10}O_5$), rhein ($C_{15}H_8O_6$), emodin ($C_{15}H_{10}O_5$), chrysophanol ($C_{15}H_{10}O_4$) and physcion ($C_{16}H_{12}O_5$), calculated with reference to the dried drug.

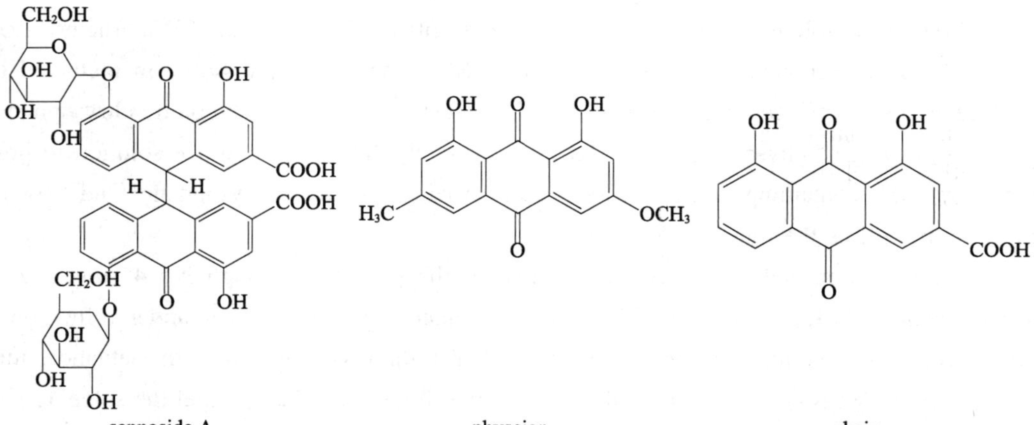

sennoside A   physcion   rhein

3. Physical and chemical properties

(1) Rhein ($C_{15}H_8O_6$): The molecular weight is 284.21; yellow needle crystal (chlor-

oform); the melting point is 321 ~ 322℃; UVλ_{Max}^{MeOH}nm: 229, 258, 435; it is soluble in alkali while it is almost insoluble in water, in addition, it is slightly soluble in ethanol, benzene, chloroform, ether and petroleum ether.

(2) Physcion ($C_{16}H_{12}O_5$): The molecular weight is 284. 26; brick red monoclinic needle crystal (benzene); the melting point is 203 ~ 207℃; UVλ_{Max}^{EtOH}nm: 266, 255, 267, 288, 440; it is insoluble in methanol, ethanol, ether and acetone, while it is soluble in alkali, benzene, chloroform and toluene.

4. Actions and indications To remove accumulation with purgation, clear *heat* and purge *fire*, cool the blood and remove toxin, expel stasis to unblock the meridian, drain dampness to abate jaundice. Accumulation, stagnation and constipation caused by excess *heat*, hematemesis caused by blood heat, red eyes and swollen throat, swelling abscess, deep - rooted boil and sore, abdominal pain caused by intestinal abscess, blood - stasis amenorrhea, postpartum stasis and obstruction, injuries from falls and fights, dampness - heat dysentery, jaundice and read urine, stranguria, edema; topical application for burn and scald. Wine - fried Rhei Radix et Rhizoma is good at clearing *heat* toxin in the upper energizer blood aspect, which can be applied for red eyes, swollen throat, painful swollen gum. The purgation power of prepared Rhei Radix et Rhizoma is mild, and it can purge *fire* and remove toxin to treat sore and ulcer caused by fire - toxin. Charred Rhei Radix et Rhizoma can cool the blood. Resolve stasis and stanch bleeding which can be applied to bleeding symptoms caused by blood *heat* and stasis.

实验二 丹参中菲醌类化合物的定性定量分析

【实验目的】

1. 掌握高效液相色谱法在醌类化合物含量测定中的应用。
2. 了解菲醌类成分的性质及其定性定量方法。

【实验原理】

同类成分结构相似，它们在检测器上的响应具有内在函数关系。一测多评法（Quantitative analysis of multi - components by single - maker, QAMS）以药材中某一成分为标准，通过其换算系数（校正因子），计算其含量，达到采用一个对照品同时测定同类其他多个成分含量的目的。

在一定范围（线性范围）内，成分的量（质量或浓度）与检测器响应成正比，即：$W = fA$，可得响应因子 $f = \frac{W}{A}$。

在丹参中丹参酮类成分多指标质量评价时，以药材中丹参酮ⅡA为参照，建立其与丹参酮Ⅰ和隐丹参酮之间的定量校正因子，通过定量校正因子计算丹参酮ⅡA、丹参酮Ⅰ和隐丹参酮总量。定量校正因子 $f_{k/m}$ 定义如下：

$$f_{k/m} = \frac{f_k}{f_m} = \frac{W_k A_m}{W_m A_k}$$

由此可导出定量计算公式：

$$W_m = \frac{W_k A_m}{f_{k/m} A_k}$$

式中 A_k 为参照物峰面积，W_k 为参照物的质量。A_m 为其他组分 m 的峰面积；W_m 为其他组分 m 的质量。

【实验器材】

1. 仪器 高效液相色谱仪，三用紫外仪，水浴锅，移液管，容量瓶，锥形瓶，量筒，展开缸。

2. 试药与试剂 丹参药材，丹参酮ⅡA，硅胶 G 薄层板，甲醇，水，乙酸乙酯，石油醚，乙醚。

【实验步骤】

1. 定性分析 取本品粉末 1g，加乙醚 5ml，振摇，放置 1 小时，滤过，滤液挥干，残渣加乙酸乙酯 1ml 使溶解，作为供试品溶液。另取丹参对照药材 1g，同法制成对照药材溶液。再取丹参酮ⅡA 对照品，加乙酸乙酯制成每 1ml 含 2mg 的溶液，作为对照品溶液。照薄层色谱法试验，吸取上述三种溶液各 5μl，分别点于同一硅胶 G 薄层板上，以石油醚（60～90℃）－乙酸乙酯（4∶1）为展开剂，展开，取出，晾干。供试品色谱中，在与对照药材色谱相应的位置上，显相同颜色的斑点；在与对照品色谱相应的位置上，显相同的暗红色斑点。

2. 定量分析

（1）色谱条件与系统适用性试验 用十八烷基硅烷键合硅胶为填充剂；乙腈（A）－0.02%磷酸水（B）为流动相，梯度如下：0～6 分钟，A 61%；20 分钟，A 90%；20.5 分钟，A 61%；25 分钟，A 61%；检测波长为 270nm。理论板数按丹参酮ⅡA 峰计算应不低于 60000。

（2）对照品溶液的制备 取丹参酮ⅡA 对照品适量，精密称取，置棕色量瓶中，加甲醇制成每 1ml 中含丹参酮ⅡA 20μg 的对照品溶液，即得。

（3）供试品溶液的制备 取丹参粉末 0.3g，精密称定，置具塞锥形瓶中，精密加入甲醇 50ml，密塞，称定重量，超声处理 30 分钟，放冷，密塞，称定重量，用甲醇补足减失的重量，摇匀，滤过，取续滤液，即得。

（4）测定法 分别精密吸取对照品溶液与供试品溶液各 10μl，注入液相色谱仪，测定；以丹参酮ⅡA 对照品为参照，以其相应的峰为 S 峰，计算丹参酮Ⅰ和隐丹参酮的相对保留时间，其相对保留时间应在规定值的 3%之内，相对保留时间及相对保留因子如下表：

待测成分（峰）	相对保留时间	校正因子
隐丹参酮	0.75	1.18
丹参酮Ⅰ	0.79	1.31
丹参酮ⅡA	1.00	1.00

以丹参酮ⅡA 的峰面积为对照，分别乘以校正因子，计算丹参酮Ⅰ、隐丹参酮、丹参酮ⅡA 的含量。

本品含丹参酮ⅡA（$C_{19}H_{18}O_3$）、丹参酮Ⅰ（$C_{18}H_{12}O_3$）和隐丹参酮（$C_{19}H_{20}O_3$）总量不得少于0.25%。

【实验记录】

1. 绘制定性薄层图，计算丹参薄层色谱图中主要斑点的R_f值。

2. HPLC法中，计算丹参中丹参酮类成分的总含量。

【思考题】

简述丹参中脂溶性成分与水溶性成分的药理作用及含量测定方法。

【相关资料】

1. 药材来源　丹参为唇形科鼠尾草属植物丹参 *Salvia miltiorrhiza* Bunge 的干燥根和根茎。春、秋二季采挖，除去泥沙，干燥。

2. 化学成分　丹参含酮类和酚类成分，脂溶性酮类成分有丹参酮ⅡA、隐丹参酮、丹参酮Ⅰ，丹参新酮；水溶性酚类成分有原儿茶醛、丹参素、丹参酚酸B等。

2015版《中国药典》规定含丹参酮ⅡA（$C_{19}H_{18}O_3$）、丹参酮Ⅰ（$C_{18}H_{12}O_3$）和隐丹参酮（$C_{19}H_{20}O_3$）总量不得少于0.25%。

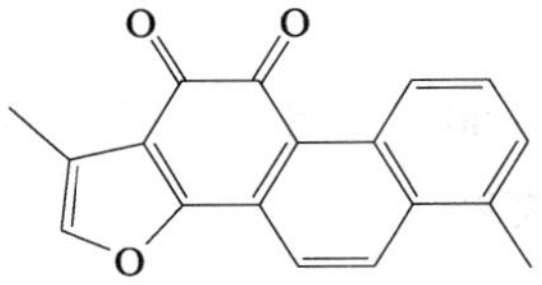

丹参酮Ⅰ

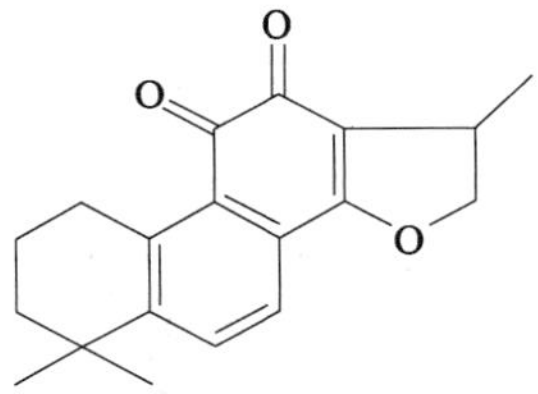

隐丹参酮

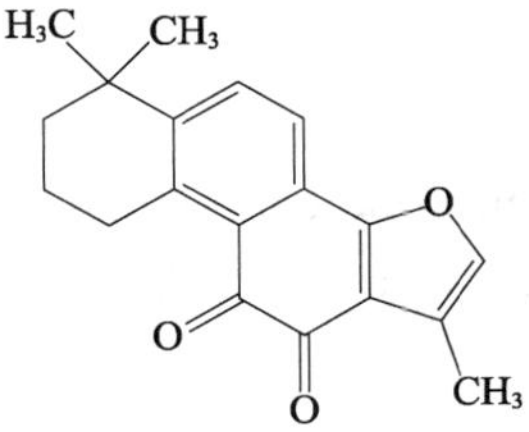

丹参酮ⅡA

3. 理化性质　丹参酮ⅡA（$C_{19}H_{18}O_3$）：分子量为294.33。樱红色针状结晶（甲醇），熔点209~210℃。不溶于水，溶于醇或其他有机溶剂。

4. 功效主治　活血祛瘀，通经止痛，清心除烦，凉血消痈。用于胸痹心痛，脘腹胁痛，癥瘕积聚，热痹疼痛，心烦不眠，月经不调，痛经经闭，疮疡肿痛。

Experiment 2　The Qualitative and Quantitative Analysis of Phenanthrene Quinone Constituents in Salvia Miltiorrhiza Radix et Rhizoma

Purpose

1. Comprehend the application of HPLC in the determination of anthraquinone compounds.

2. Know about the properties of phenanthrenequinone and their qualitative and quantitative methods.

Principle

In recent years, the quantitative analysis of multiple major components in traditional

Chinese medicines (TCMs) has been considered as an effective approach for quality control purposes. However, this approach has been limited due to the need for high - purity (98%) commercial standard substances. To solve this problem, a method that uses single standard substances for the quantitative analysis of multi - component (termed quantitative analysis of multi - component with single marker, or QAMS) in TCMs was established and has been adopted in Chinese Pharmacopoeia. The detector responses of compounds with similar structures have functional relationships. The standard substance of which is inexpensive and can easily be obtained is selected as the internal referring substance. The concentration of the internal referring substance in the herb is determined by external standard method, whereas the concentrations of other analytes in the herb are calculated with their relative correction factors and their peak areas.

The detector response has linear relationship with the levels of components within certain concentration ranges. That is $W = fA$.

The relative correction factors of analytes are calculated using the standard substance according to equation (1).

$$f_{k/m} = \frac{f_k}{f_m} = \frac{W_k A_m}{W_m A_k} \qquad (1)$$

Thus, the concentrations of other analytes in the herb are calculated according to equation (2) with their relative correction factors and their peak areas.

$$W_m = \frac{W_k A_m}{f_{k/m} A_k} \qquad (2)$$

Where A_k *and* A_m represent the peak areas of internal referring substance and the analyte, respectively, and W_k and W_m represent the concentrations of internal referring substance and the analyte.

Conditions

1. Apparatus HPLC instrument, ultraviolet analyzer, water bath, pipette, volumetric flask, conical flask, graduated cylinder and expansion cylinder.

2. Reagents and materials Salvia Miltiorrhiza Radix et Rhizoma, tanshinone IIA, Silica gel G thin layer plate, methanol, water, ethyl acetate, petroleum ether and ethyl ether.

Experimental Procedure

1. Qualitative analysis Shake 1g of the powder with 5ml of ether, stand for 1 hour and filter. Evaporate the filtrate to dryness, dissolve the residue in 1ml of ethyl acetate as the test solution. Prepare a solution of Salviae Miltiorrhizae Radix et Rhizoma reference drug in the same manner as the reference drug solution. Dissolve Tanshinone ⅡA CRS in ethyl acetate to produce a solution of 2mg per ml as the reference solution. Carry out the method for thin layer chromatography, using silica gel G as the coating substance and a mixture of petroleum ether (60 ~ 90℃) and ethyl acetate (4:1) as the mobile phase. Apply separately 5μl of each of the three solutions to the plate. After developing and removal of the plate, dry in air. The spots in the chromatogram obtained with the test solution correspond in position and colour to the spots in the chromatogram obtained with the reference drug solution; and a dark

– red spot in the chromatogram obtained with the test solution corresponds in position and colour to the spot in the chromatogram obtained with the reference solution.

2. Quantitative analysis

(1) Chromatographic system and system suitability　Use octadectylsilane bonded silica gel as the stationary phase, acetonitrile as the mobile phase A and 0.02% phosphoric acid as the mobile phase B, elute in gradient as following: 0 ~ 6min, A 61%; 20min, A 90%; 20.5min, A 61%; 25min, A 61%; As detector a spectrophotometer set at 270nm. The flow rate is 1.0ml/min. The number of theoretical plates of the column is not less than 60000, calculated with the reference to the peak of tanshinone ⅡA.

(2) Reference solution　Weigh accurately a quantity of tanshinone ⅡA CRS to an amber volumetric flask, dissolve in methanol to prepare a solution containing 20μg per ml as the reference solution.

(3) Test solution　Weigh accurately 0.3g of the powder (through a No. 3 sieve) to a stopper conical flask. Add accurately 50ml of methanol, and weigh. Ultrasonicate (power 250W, frequency 33 kHz) for 30 minutes, cool and weigh again, replenish the loss of weight with methanol, mix well and filter, use the successive filtrate as the test solution.

(4) Procedure　Accurately inject 10μl of each of the reference solution and the test solution, respectively, into the column. The relative retention time of cryptotanshinone and tanshinone Ⅰ against tanshinone ⅡA were calculated. The variation of the relative retention time should be within ±3%. The relative retention time and the relative correction factors of cryptotanshinone, tanshinone I and tanshinone ⅡA are as follows:

Analytes	relative retention time	relative correction factors
Cryptotanshinone	0.75	1.18
tanshinone Ⅰ	0.79	1.31
tanshinone ⅡA	1.00	1.00

The concentrations of cryptotanshinone, tanshinone Ⅰ and tanshinone ⅡA in the herb are calculated with their relative correction factors and their peak areas.

Experimental Records

1. Draw the chromatogram of thin layer chromatography and calculate R_f values of cryptotanshinone and tanshinone ⅡA.

2. Calculate the content of tanshinone by external method.

Questions

Describe the pharmacological effects and the analysis of liposoluble and water – soluble component in Salvia Miltiorrhiza Radix et Rhizoma.

Background Information

1. Origins　*Salvia Miltiorrhiza* Radix et Rhizoma is the dried root and rhizome of *Salvia miltiorrhiza* Bge. (Fam. Labiatae). The drug is collected in spring or autumn. Removed from soil, and dried.

2. Chemical constituents Salvia Miltiorrhiza Radix et Rhizoma mainly contains lipophilic diterpenoid quinones and hydrophilic phenolic acid. The quniones maily include tanshinone ⅡA, cryptotanshinone, tanshinone Ⅰ, miltirone and so on. The phenolic acid compounds mainly include protocatechuic aldehyde, danshensu, salvianolic acid B and so on.

In People′s Republic of China Pharmacopoeia (2015 edition), it contains not less than 0.25 percent of cryptotanshinone, tanshinone Ⅰ and tanshinone ⅡA (by HPLC).

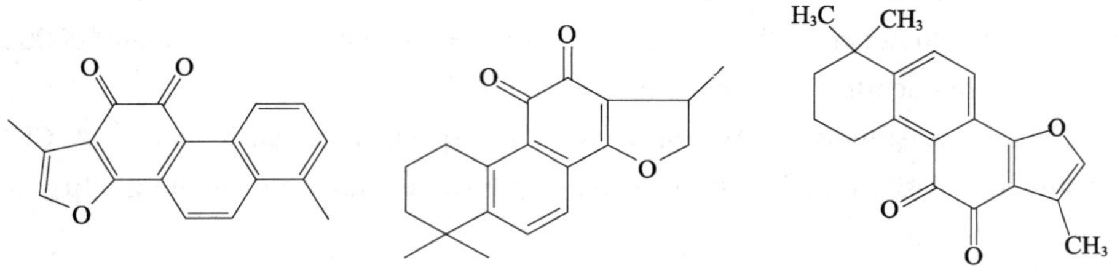

tanshinone　　cryptotanshinone　　tanshinone ⅡA

3. Physical and chemical properties Tanshinone ⅡA ($C_{19}H_{18}O_3$): The molecular weight is 294.33; cherry red needle crystal (methanol); the melting point is 209 ~ 210℃; It is insoluble in water, while it is soluble in alcohol or other organic solvents.

4. Actions and indications To activate blood and eliminate stasis, unblock the meridian to relieve pain, clear the heart and relieve vexation, cool the blood and disperse abscesses. Chest impediment and heart pain, pain in the epigastrium and abdomen, hypochondriac pain, aggregation and accumulation, painful heat impediment, insomnia caused by vexation, menstrual irregularitiets, dysmenorrhea and amenorrhea, sore, ulcer, swelling and pain.

实验三　紫草中萘醌类化合物的定性定量分析

【实验目的】

了解萘醌成分的性质，掌握紫草的定性、定量原理及操作。

【实验原理】

1. 紫外分光光度法　紫草中主要含有萘醌类化合物。萘醌类化合物具有较高的共轭结构，因而具有紫外吸收。紫草中相对含量较高的化合物紫草素的最大吸收波长与总萘醌的最大吸收波长一致，因此可以用紫草素为对照，测定总萘醌类化合物的含量。

2. 高效液相色谱法　本实验采用高效液相色谱法，以β，β′-二甲基丙烯酰阿卡宁为对照品，在与对照相同的保留时间处确定样品中β，β′-二甲基丙烯酰阿卡宁的峰位置，并测定其峰面积，用外标一点法计算其含量。

【实验器材】

1. 仪器　高效液相色谱仪，三用紫外分析仪，超声仪，移液管，容量瓶，锥形瓶，量筒，展开缸。

2. 试药与试剂　紫草药材，左旋紫草素对照品，β，β′-二甲基丙烯酰阿卡宁对照品，硅胶G薄层板，环己烷，甲苯，水，乙酸乙酯，石油醚，甲酸，乙醇，乙腈。

【实验步骤】

1. 定性分析 取本品粉末0.5g，加石油醚（60~90℃）20ml，超声处理20分钟，滤过，滤液浓缩至1ml，作为供试品溶液。另取紫草对照药材0.5g，同法制成对照药材溶液。照薄层色谱法试验，吸取上述两种溶液各4μl，分别点于同一硅胶G薄层板上，以环己烷-甲苯-乙酸乙酯-甲酸（5∶5∶0.5∶0.1）为展开剂，展开，取出，晾干。供试品色谱中，在与对照药材色谱相应的位置上，显相同的紫红色斑点；再喷以10%氢氧化钾甲醇溶液，斑点变为蓝色。

2. 定量分析

（1）紫外分光光度法测定紫草中羟基萘醌总色素的含量　取本品适量，在50℃干燥3小时，粉碎（过三号筛），取约0.5g，精密称定，置100ml量瓶中，加乙醇至刻度，4小时内时时振摇，滤过。精密量取续滤液5ml，置25ml量瓶中，加乙醇至刻度，摇匀。照紫外-可见分光光度法，在516nm波长处测定吸光度，按左旋紫草素（$C_{16}H_{16}O_5$）的吸收系数为242计算，即得。

（2）HPLC法测定紫草中β，β′-二甲基丙烯酰阿卡宁的含量

①色谱条件与系统适用性试验　以十八烷基硅烷键合硅胶为填充剂；以乙腈-水-甲酸（70∶30∶0.05）为流动相；流速：1.0ml/min；检测波长为275nm。理论板数按β，β′-二甲基丙烯酰阿卡宁峰计算应不低于2000。

②对照品溶液的制备　取β，β′-二甲基丙烯酰阿卡宁对照品适量，精密称定，加乙醇制成每1ml含0.1mg的溶液，即得。

③供试品溶液的制备　取本品粉末（过四号筛）约0.5g，精密称定，置具塞锥形瓶中，精密加入石油醚（60~90℃）25ml，称定重量，超声处理（功率250W，频率33kHz）30分钟，放冷，再称定重量，用石油醚（60~90℃）补足减失的亘量，摇匀，滤过。精密量取续滤液10ml，蒸干，残渣加流动相溶解，转移至10ml量瓶中，加流动相至刻度，摇匀，滤过，取续滤液，即得。

④测定法　分别精密吸取对照品溶液与供试品溶液各10μl，注入液相色谱仪，测定，即得。

【实验记录】

1. 绘制定性薄层图，计算紫草薄层色谱图中主要斑点的R_f值。
2. 绘制标准曲线，计算紫草中羟基萘醌总色素的含量。
3. HPLC法中，用外标一点法计算紫草中β，β′-二甲基丙烯酰阿卡宁的含量。

【思考题】

1. 紫外分光光度法测定紫草中紫草素类成分的优势是什么？
2. 如某一中药制剂中含有紫草，如何排除其他干扰成分对紫草素类成分含量测定的影响？

【相关资料】

1. 药材来源 本品为紫草科植物新疆紫草 *Arnebia euchroma*（Royle）Johnst. 或内蒙紫草 *Arnebia guttata* Bunge 的干燥根。春、秋二季采挖，除去泥沙，干燥。

2. 化学成分 紫草含有的多种萘醌类色素，是其有效成分。紫草素为紫草素类的

母体，多结合成酯而存在。主要成分为乙酰紫草素、β，β′-二甲基丙烯酰阿卡宁等。

2015 版《中国药典》规定本品含羟基萘醌总色素以左旋紫草素计，不得少于 0.80%（用分光光度法），含β，β′-二甲基丙烯酰阿卡宁（$C_{21}H_{22}O_6$）不得少于 0.30%（HPLC 法）。

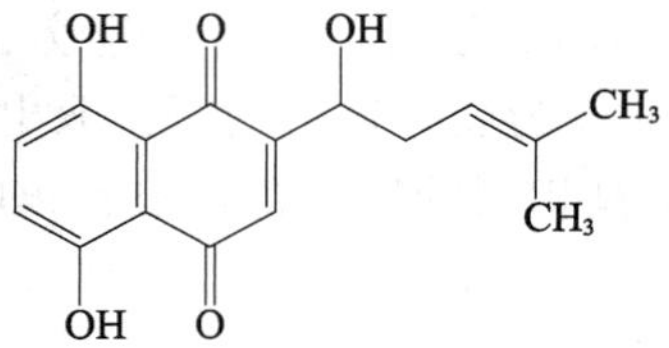

紫草素

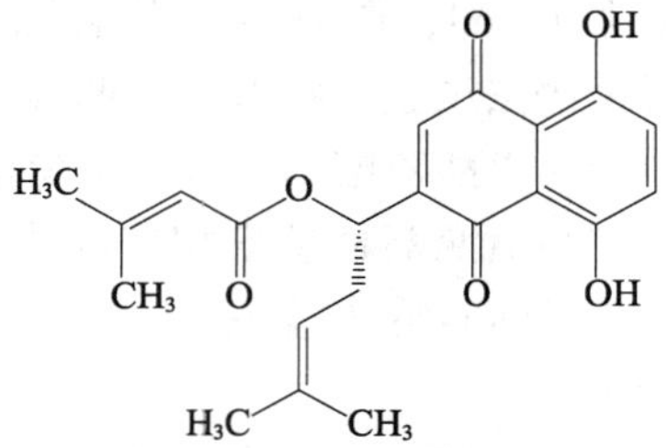

β，β′-二甲基丙烯酰阿卡宁

3. 理化性质

（1）紫草素（$C_{16}H_{16}O_5$）　分子量为 288.31。红褐色针晶（石油醚），熔点 147～149℃，$[\alpha]_D^{20}$ +138°（苯）。不溶于水，溶于醇、有机溶剂和植物油。UV $\lambda_{Max}^{CCl_4}$nm（ε）：560（5012）、543（5012）、524（7943）、488（6310）。

（2）β，β′-二甲基丙烯酰阿卡宁（$C_{21}H_{22}O_6$）　分子量为 370.40，红色板状结晶，熔点 116～117℃，旋光度 $[\alpha]_{643}$ -100°。易溶于苯、乙醚、三氯甲烷、丙酮和乙醇，微溶于热水，不溶于冷水。

4. 功效主治　清热凉血，活血解毒，透疹消斑。用于血热毒盛，斑疹紫黑，麻疹不透，疮疡，湿疹，水火烫伤。

Experiment 3　The Qualitative and Quantitative Analysis of Naphthoquinone Constituents in Arnebiae Radix

Purpose

To know about the properties of naphthoquinone and comprehend the qualitative and quantitative methods of Arnebiae Radix.

Principle

1. Ultraviolet - visible spectroscopy　The main compounds in Arnebiae Radix are naphthoquinones, which have good absorption under UV due to their highly conjugated structures. The maximum absorption of shikonin is consistent with the total naphthoquinones in Arnebiae Radix. Thus, the total naphthoquinones in Arnebiae Radix can be determined with shikonin as the reference.

2. HPLC　In this experiment, we will determine the content of β, β′ - dimethylacrylalkannin in Arnebiae Radix. We can identify the peak of β, β′ - dimethylacrylalkannin in the sample through comparing the retention time with reference. Then, the content of β, β′ - dimethylacrylalkannin in the sample can be calculated by the external standard method.

Conditions

1. Apparatus　HPLC instrument, ultraviolet analyzer, ultrasonic cleaner, pipette, volumetric flask, conical flask, graduated cylinder and expansion cylinder.

2. Reagents and materials Arnebiae Radix, Shikonin CRS, β, β′-dimethylacrylalkanin CRS, silica gel G thin layer plate, cyclohexane, toluene, water, ethyl acetate, petroleum ether, formic acid, ethanol and acetonitrile.

Experimental Procedure

1. Qualitative analysis Weigh 0.5g of the powder and add 20ml of petroleum ether (60~90℃), ultrasonicate for 20 minutes and filter. Concentrate the filtrate to about 1ml as the test solution. Prepare a solution of 0.5g of Arnebiae Radix reference drug in the same manner as the reference drug solution. Carry out the method for thin layer chromatography, using silica gel G as the coating substance and a mixture of cyclohexane, toluene, ethyl acetate and formic acid (5:5:0.5:0.1) as the mobile phase. Apply separately to the plate 4μl of each of the above two solutions. After developing and removal of the plate, dry in air. The purplish-red spots in the chromatogram obtained with the test solution correspond in position and color to the spots obtained with the reference drug solution; and the color of spots turn to blue after spraying with a 10% solution of potassium hydroxide in methanol.

2. Quantitative analysis

(1) Determination of total content of hydroxynaphthaquinone Weigh accurately 0.5g of the powder (through No. 3 sieve), previously dried at 50℃ for 3 hours, to a 100ml volumetric flask, add ethanol to volume, shake constantly for 4 hours, filter, measure accurately 5ml of the successivc filtrate to a 25ml volumetric flask, dilute with ethanol to volume and mix well. Carry out the method for ultraviolet spectrophotometry and colourimetry, measure the absorbance at 516nm, calculate the content of shikonin ($C_{16}H_{16}O_5$), taking 242 as the value of absorption coefficient (1%, 1cm). It contains not less than 0.80 percent of total pigments of hydroxynaphthaquinone, calculated as shikonin ($C_{16}H_{16}O_5$) with reference to the dried drug.

(2) Determination of β, β′-dimethylacrylalkanin in Arnebiae Radix by HPLC

①Chromatographic system and system suitability Use octadecylsilane bonded silica gel as the stationary phase and a mixture of acetonitrile, water and formic acid (70:30:0.05) as the mobile phase. The flow rate is 1.0ml/min. As detector a spectrophotometer set at 275nm. The number of theoretical plates of the column is not less than 2000, calculated with reference to the peak of β, β′-dimethylacrylalkanin.

②Reference solution Weigh accurately a quantity of β, β′-dimethylacrylalkanin CRS, dissolve in ethanol to produce a solution containing 0.1mg per ml.

③Test solution Weigh accurately 0.5g of the powder (through No. 4 sieve) to a stopper conical flask. Add accurately 25ml of petroleum ether (60~90℃), and weigh. Ultrasonicate (power 250W, frequency 33kHz) for 30 minutes, cool and weigh again, replenish the loss of solvent with petroleum ether (60~90℃), mix well and filter. Measure accurately 10ml of the successive filtrate, evaporate to dryness, dissolve the residue with the mobile phase and transfer to a 10ml volumetric flask, dilute to volume with the mobile phase and mix well.

④Procedure Inject accurately 10μl of each of the reference solution and the test solution, respectively, into the column, determine and calculate the content.

Experimental Records

1. Draw the chromatogram of thin layer chromatography, calculate R_f values of the main components.

2. Plot the standard curve, and calculate the content of total hydroxylnaphthoquinone in Arnebiae Radix.

3. After the determination, calculate the content of β, β′ - dimethylacrylalkanin in Arnebiae Radix by external standard method.

Questions

1. What is the advantage of UV spectrophotometry in the assay of shikonin in Arnebiae Radix?

2. How to eliminate the influence of interfering components in the determination of shikonin in traditional Chinese preparation?

Background Information

1. Origins Arnebia Root is the dried root of *Arnebia euchroma* (Royle) Johnst, or *Arnebia guttata* Bunge (Fam. Boraginaceae). The drug is collected in spring or autumn, removed from soil, and dried.

2. Chemical constituents Naphthoquinones are the main bioactive components in Arnebiae Radix. Shikonin is often combined into ester. The main ingredients are acethlshikonin and β, β′ - dimethylacrylalkanin and so on.

In People′s Republic of China Pharmacopoeia (2015 edition), it should contain not less than 0.80 percent of total pigments of hydroxynaphthaquinone, calculated as shikonin ($C_{16}H_{16}O_5$) with reference to the dried drug (by spectrophotometry), and it contains not less than 0.30 percent of β, β′ - dimethylacrylalkanin ($C_{16}H_{16}O_5$) (by HPLC).

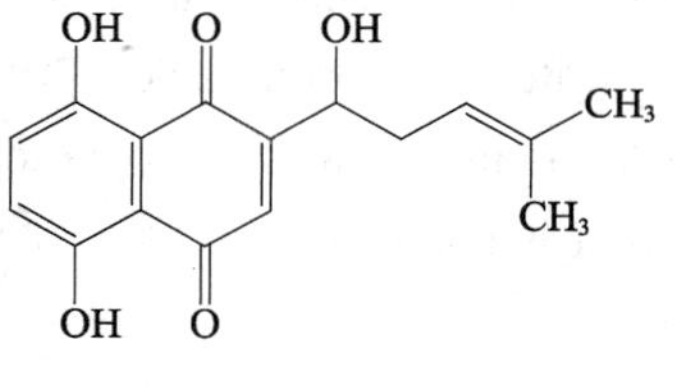

shikonin

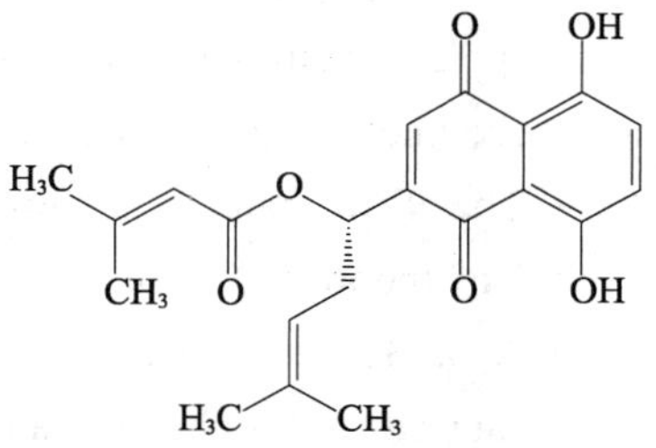

β, β′-dimethylacrylalkanin

3. Physical and chemical properties

(1) Shikonin ($C_{16}H_{16}O_5$) The molecular weight is 288.31; reddish - brown needle crystal (petroleum ether); the melting point is 147 ~ 149℃; $[\alpha]_D^{20}$ +138° (Benzene); UV $\lambda_{Max}^{CCl_4}$nm (ε): 560 (5012), 543 (5012), 524 (7943), 488 (6310); It is insoluble in water, soluble in alcohol, organic solvents and vegetable oils.

(2) β, β′ - dimethylacrylalkanin ($C_{16}H_{16}O_5$) The molecular weight is 370.4; red

plate crystal; the melting point is 116 ~ 117℃; $[\alpha]_{643}$ −100°; it is soluble in benzene, ethyl ether, chloroform, acetone and ethanol while it is slightly soluble in water and insoluble in cold water.

4. Actions and indications To clear heat and cool the blood, activate blood and remove toxin, promote eruption to resolve macule. Exuberant blood heat – toxin, dark purple macule and papule, unerupted measles, sore and ulcer, eczema, scald and burn.

实验四　三黄片中蒽醌类化合物的定性定量分析

【实验目的】

掌握中药复方制剂中蒽醌类成分的主要定性、定量分析方法。

【实验原理】

三黄片主要由大黄300g，盐酸小檗碱5g，黄芩浸膏21g制成，是一种具有清热泻火、消炎利便功效的常见中成药。大黄为方中主药，主要有效成分为芦荟大黄素、大黄酸、大黄素、大黄酚、大黄素甲醚蒽醌衍生物，以部分游离、大部分与葡萄糖结合成苷的形式存在，约占大黄成分的3% ~5%。这类化合物具有很强的共轭结构，通常具有紫外吸收，因而在薄层色谱法中可置于紫外灯下进行斑点的定位，高效液相色谱法中也可用紫外检测器进行含量测定。蒽醌苷类成分在酸性条件下加热易水解为所对应的苷元，根据苷元类成分易溶于小极性的有机溶剂的性质，可实现与其他类型成分的分离。

【实验器材】

1. 仪器　高效液相色谱仪，三用紫外分析仪，超声仪，水浴锅。

2. 试药与试剂　三黄片，大黄对照药材，大黄素对照品，大黄酚对照品，硅胶G板，环己烷，乙酸乙酯，甲酸，乙醇，三氯甲烷，水，10%三氯化铝乙醇，甲醇，磷酸。

【实验步骤】

1. 定性分析　取本品5片，除去包衣，研细，取约0.25g，加甲醇5ml，超声处理5分钟，滤过，滤液作为供试品溶液。另取大黄对照药材0.2g，加甲醇3ml，同法制成对照药材溶液。照薄层色谱法试验，吸取上述两种溶液各5μl，分别点于同一以羧甲基纤维素钠为黏合剂的硅胶G薄层板上，以环己烷－乙酸乙酯－甲酸（12∶3∶0.1）作为展开剂，展开，取出，晾干，置紫外光灯（365nm）下检视。供试品色谱中，在与对照药材色谱相应的位置上，显相同的荧光斑点。

2. 定量分析

（1）色谱条件与系统适用性试验　以十八烷基键合硅胶为填充剂；以甲醇－0.1%磷酸（85∶15）为流动相；流速：1.0ml/min；检测波长为254nm。理论塔板数按大黄素峰计算应不低于2000。

（2）对照品溶液的制备　取大黄素对照品、大黄酚对照品适量，精密称定，分别加无水乙醇－乙酸乙酯（2∶1）制成每1ml含大黄素10μg的溶液和每1ml含大黄酚

25μg 的溶液，即得。

（3）供试品溶液的制备　取本品 20 片，除去包衣，研细（过三号筛），取约 0.26g，精密称定，精密加入乙醇 25ml，称定重量，加热回流 1 小时，放冷，用乙醇补足减失的重量，摇匀，滤过，精密量取续滤液 10ml，置烧瓶中，蒸干，加 30% 乙醇 - 盐酸（10∶1）的混合液 15ml，置水浴中加热回流 1 小时，立即冷却，用三氯甲烷萃取 4 次，每次 15ml，合并三氯甲烷溶液，转移至 25ml 量瓶中，并稀释至刻度，摇匀，滤过，取续滤液，即得。

（4）测定法　分别精密吸取对照品溶液与供试品溶液各 10μl，注入液相色谱仪，测定，即得。

【实验记录】

1. 绘制定性薄层图，计算三黄片薄层色谱图中主要斑点的 R_f 值。
2. 用外标一点法计算三黄片中大黄素（$C_{15}H_{10}O_5$）和大黄酚（$C_{25}H_{10}O_4$）的总量。

【思考题】

1. 用 30% 乙醇 - 盐酸（10∶1）的混合液，置水浴中加热回流的目的是什么？
2. 若要测定三黄片中小檗碱的含量，请设计定性定量方法。

【相关资料】

1. 处方、制法及药材来源　三黄片主要由大黄 300g，盐酸小檗碱 5g，黄芩浸膏 21g 制成。以上三味，黄芩浸膏系取黄芩，加水煎煮三次，第一次 1.5 小时；第二次 1 小时；第三次 40 分钟；合并煎液，滤过，滤液用盐酸调节 pH 值至 1 ~ 2，静置 1 小时，取沉淀，用水洗涤使 pH 值至 5 ~ 7，烘干，粉碎成细粉。取大黄 150g，碎成细粉，剩余大黄粉碎成粗粉，用 30% 乙醇回流提取三次，滤过，合并滤液，回收乙醇并减压浓缩成稠膏，加入大黄细粉、盐酸小檗碱细粉、黄芩浸膏细粉及适量辅料，混匀，制成颗粒，干燥，压制成 1000 片，包衣，即得。本品为糖衣或薄膜衣片，除去包衣后显棕色；味苦、微涩。

2. 功效主治　清热解毒，泻火通便。用于三焦热盛所致的目赤肿痛、口鼻生疮、咽喉肿痛、牙龈肿痛、心烦口渴、尿黄便秘；也用于急性胃肠炎，痢疾。

3. 化学成分及理化性质　见本章实验一。

（杨杰）

Experiment 4　The Qualitative and Quantitative Analysis of Anthraquinone Constituents in Sanhuang Tablets

Purpose

Comprehend the main methods for qualitative and quantitative analysis of anthraquinone compounds in Traditional Chinese Medicine preparation.

Principle

SanHuang Tablets is a traditional Chinese preparation used for clearing heat, removing toxin, purging *fire* and relaxing the bowels. It is composed of Rhei Radix et Rhizoma, extract of Scutellariae Radix and berberine. The main drug in this preparation is Rhei Radix et Rhizoma which contains anthraquinones such as rhein, emodin, chrysophanol. They exist in the free form or glycoside. The content of anthraquinones in Rhei Radix et Rhizoma is about 3% ~5%. Therefore, the content of anthraquinones is highly related to the quality of this preparation. Anthraquinones usually have good absorption under UV due to their highly conjugated structures. So the spots of compounds can be seen by illuminating the TLC plate with short - wave UV and these compounds can be easily detected by UV detector in HPLC. In this experiment, glycosides of anthraquinones are acid hydrolyzed into their corresponding aglycones, which are further extracted with chloroform.

Conditions

1. Apparatus HPLC instrument, ultraviolet visible spectrophotometer, ultraviolet analyzer, ultrasonic cleaner and water bath.

2. Reagents and materials Sanhuang Tablets, Rhei Radix et Rhizoma CRS, emodin CRS, chrysophanol CRS, silica gel G thin layer plate, cyclohexane, ethyl acetate, formic acid, ethanol, chloroform, water, 10% aluminum chloride, ethanol, methanol and phosphoric acid.

Experimental Procedure

1. Qualitative analysis Pulverize 5 tablets, with coating removed. To 0.25g, add 5ml of methanol, ultrasonicate for 5 minutes, filter and use the filtrate as the test solution. To 0.2g of Rhei Radix et Rhizoma reference drug, add 3ml of methanol, ultrasonicate for 5 minutes and use the supernatant as the reference drug solution. Carry out the method for thin layer chromatography, using silica gel G as the coating substance and a mixture of cyclohexane, ethyl acetate, formic acid (12∶3∶0.1) as the mobile phase. Apply separately 5μl of each of the two solutions to the plate. After developing and removal of the plate, dry in air. Examine under ultraviolet light at 365nm. The fluorescent spots in the chromatogram obtained with the test solution correspond in position and color to the spots in the chromatogram obtained with the reference drug solution.

2. Quantitative analysis

(1) Chromatographic system and system suitability　Use octadecylsilane bonded silica gel as the stationary phase and a mixture of methanol and 0.1% solution of phosphoric acid (85∶15) as the mobile phase. The flow rate is 1.0ml/min. As detector a spectrophotometer set at 254nm. The number of the theoretical plates of the column is not less than 2000, calculated with reference to the peak of emodin.

(2) Reference solution　Dissolve a quantity of emodin CRS and chrysophanol CRS, accurately weighed, in a mixture of dehydrated ethanol and ethyl acetate (2∶1) to produce a solution containing 10μg emodin and 25μg of chrysophanol per ml as the reference solution.

(3) Test solution　Weigh accurately 20 tablets, removed the coats, and pulverize to fine powder. Weigh accurately 0.2g of the powder (through No. 3 sieve) in a conical flask,

add accurately 25ml of ethanol, stopper closely and weigh. Heat under refulx on a water bath for 1 hour, allow it to cool, replenish the loss of solvent with ethanol, shake well, filter, and discard the initial filtrate. Transfer accurately 10ml of the successive filtrate to a flask, evaporate to dryness. Heat and hydrolyze the residue with 15ml of a mixture of 30% ethanol and hydrochloric acid (10∶1) on a water bath for 1 hour, cool immediately, extract with four 15ml quantities of chloroform, combine the chloroform extract, evaporate to dryness. Dissolve the residue in a mixture of dehydrated ethanol and ethyl acetate (2∶1), transfer to a 25ml volumetric flask, dilute to volume, mix well and filter. Discard the initial filtrate and use the successive filtrate as the test solution.

(4) Procedure Inject accurately 10μl of each of the reference solution and the test solution, into the column, determine and calculate the content.

Experimental Records

1. Draw the chromatogram of thin layer chromatography and calculate R_f values of main components in Sanhuang tablets.

2. Calculate the total contents of emodin and chrysophanol by external standard method.

Questions

1. What is the purpose of using a mixture of 30% ethanol and hydrochloric acid (10∶1) on a water bath for 1 hour?

2. To determine the content of berberine in Sanhuang Tablets, please design a qualitative and quantitative method.

Background Information

1. Ingredients and Procedure Rhei Radix et Rhizoma 300g; Berberine Hydrochloride 5g; Scutellariae Extract 21g. Scutellariae Extract is the extract from Scutellariae Radix. Decoct Scutellariae Radix with water for 3 times, 1. 5 hours for the first time, 1 hour for the second time and 40 minutes for the third time, respectively, combine the decoctions and filter. Adjust the filter to pH 5 ~ 7, heat to dryness and pulverize to fine powder. Pulverize 150g of Rhei Radix et Rhizoma to fine powder. Heat under refulx the rest of Rhei Radix et Rhizoma, in coarse powder, with 30% ethanol for 3 times, filter, combine the filtrate, recover ethanol and concentrate on vacuum to a thick extract. Add the fine powder of Rhei Radix et Rhizoma, berberine hydrochloride, Scutellariae Extract and a quantity of excipient, mix thoroughly, make granules, dry, and compress into 1000 tablets and coat with sugar or film. Sugar coated or film coated tablets with brown core taste, bitter and slightly astringent.

2. The chemicalconstituents and physicochemical properties of Rhei Radix et Rhizoma see Experiment 1 of this chapter.

3. Actions and indications To clear *heat*, remove toxin, purge *fire* and relax the bowels. Red painful swelling eyes, throat and gums, mouth and nose sores, vexation thirst yellow urine, and constipation, which are caused by exuberant heat in triple energizer.

(Jie Yang)

第四章
皂苷类成分的分析

实验一　柴胡中皂苷类成分的定性定量分析

【实验目的】

1. 掌握可见 - 紫外分光光度法的原理及操作。
2. 熟悉分光光度法在测定皂苷类药物中的应用。

【实验原理】

有色溶液对不同波长的入射光有不同程度的吸收，每种物质都有其特定的吸收光谱。有些无色溶液可通过化学反应生成有色物质。溶液颜色的深浅往往是溶液浓度高低的标志，而颜色的深浅与对一定波长光的吸收度有关。因此，可通过比较溶液的吸收度来测定溶液中物质的含量。

【实验器材】

1. 仪器　电子天平，超声仪，可见 - 紫外分光光度计，具塞锥形瓶，旋转蒸发仪，硅胶 G 薄层板，毛细管，量瓶，三用紫外分析仪。

2. 试药与试剂　柴胡皂苷 d 对照品，柴胡药材粉末，氨水，甲醇，正丁醇，三氯甲烷，乙酸乙酯，2% 对二甲氨基苯甲醛的 40% 硫酸溶液，1% 对二甲氨基苯甲醛的乙醇溶液，磷酸。

【实验步骤】

1. 定性分析　取柴胡样品粉末（过四号筛）0.5g，精密称定，置具塞锥形瓶中，加入含 5% 浓氨水试液的甲醇溶液 25ml，密塞，超声处理 30 分钟，滤过，用甲醇分 2 次洗涤容器及药渣，洗液与滤液合并，回收溶剂至干。残渣加少量水溶解，再用水饱和的正丁醇提取 3 次，每次 20ml，合并正丁醇液，用水洗涤 2 次，每次 20ml，弃去水液，回收正丁醇至干，加甲醇溶解、定容至 5ml，摇匀，作为供试品溶液。另取柴胡皂苷 d 对照品适量，分别加甲醇制成每 1ml 含 0.2mg 的溶液，作为对照品溶液。吸取上述溶液各 4μl，分别点于同一硅胶 G 薄层板上，以三氯甲烷 - 乙酸乙酯 - 甲醇 - 水（15:40:22:10）（10℃以下放置的下层溶液）为展开剂，展开，取出，晾干，喷以 2% 对二甲氨基苯甲醛的 40% 硫酸溶液，在 60℃加热至斑点显色清晰，分别置日光和紫外光灯（365nm）下检视。供试品色谱中，在与对照品色谱相应的位置上，应显相同的黄色荧光斑点。

2. 定量分析

（1）供试品溶液的制备　按定性分析项下供试品溶液的制备方法制备。

（2）对照品溶液的制备　精密称取柴胡皂苷 d 对照品适量，加甲醇制成每 1ml 含 1mg 的溶液，即得。

（3）标准曲线的制备　分别精密量取对照品溶液 0.2、0.4、0.6、0.8、1.0ml 置 1ml 量瓶中，加甲醇定容至刻度，摇匀。精密吸取各对照品溶液 0.2ml，置 10ml 具塞试管中，分别加入 1% 对二甲氨基苯甲醛乙醇溶液 0.1ml，70℃温热 10 分钟，取出放冷，加入磷酸 4.0ml，70℃反应 30min，放冷，在波长 545nm 处分别测定各对照品溶液的吸光度值。以柴胡皂苷 d 质量为横坐标（x），吸光度值为纵坐标（y），绘制标准曲线，得回归方程。

（4）样品测定　精密吸取供试品溶液 0.2ml，按标准曲线项下方法操作，在波长 545nm 处测定供试品溶液的吸光度值，由标准曲线计算含量。

【实验记录】

1. 简述操作过程，记录实验现象。
2. 绘制定性层析图谱，算出主要斑点的 R_f 值。
3. 绘制标准曲线，计算回归方程与相关系数。
4. 计算柴胡中总皂苷的含量。

【思考题】

1. 进行定量分析时，皂苷类成分还可用哪些显色剂显色？
2. 请设计另一方案，定性鉴别柴胡药材。

【相关资料】

1. 药材来源　柴胡为伞形科植物柴胡 *Bupleurum chinense* DC. 或狭叶柴胡 *Bupleurum scorzonerifolium* Willd. 的干燥根。

2. 主要化学成分　柴胡主要含有皂苷、黄酮、挥发油、香豆素、甾醇、多糖等成分。其中皂苷类成分主要有柴胡皂苷 a、b、c、d（saikosaponins a，b，c，d）等。柴胡皂苷 d 为白色粉末，分子量 780.98，分子式 $C_{42}H_{68}O_{13}$，熔点 212～218℃，无紫外吸收。

3. 功能与主治　柴胡具有和解表里，疏肝，升阳的功效。常用于感冒发热，寒热往来，胸胁胀痛，月经不调，子宫脱垂，脱肛等症。

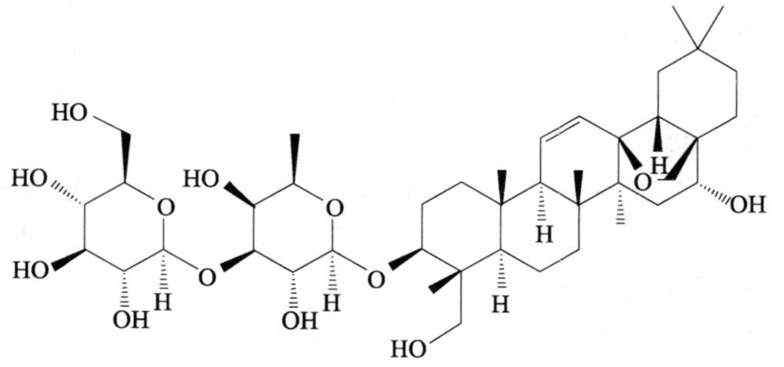

柴胡皂苷d

Experiment 1　The Qualitative and Quantitative Analysis of Saponins in Bupleuri Radix

Purpose

1. Comprehend the application of spectrophotometry in analysis of saponin.

2. Understand the principle and operation of ultraviolet – visible spectrophotometry.

Principle

Solution of colored substance can absorb beam of different wavelength in different degree. Each substance has its specific absorption spectrum. Some colorless solution can generate a color substance by a chemistry reaction. The color depth is often a sign of the solution's concentration, which depends on the absorption of a certain wavelength. For the reason, we can determinate the content of substance in solution by the means of comparing the absorbency of the solution.

Condition

1. Apparatus　Electronic balance, ultrasonic cleaner, ultraviolet – visible spectrophotometer, stopper conical flask, rotary evaporator, silica gel G plate, capillaries, volumetric flask and ultraviolet analyzer.

2. Reagents and Materials　Ammonia water, methanol, *n* – butanol, chloroform, ethyl acetate, 2% solution of *p* – dimethylaminobenzaldehyde in 40% sulfuric acid solution, 1% solution of *p* – dimethylaminobenzaldehyde in ethanol solution, phosphoric acid, saikosaponind CRS and Radix Bupleuri powder.

Experimental Procedure

1. Qualitative analysis　Weigh accurately 0. 5g of the powder to a stoppered conical flash, add 25ml of methanol solution with 5% ammonia water, ultrasonicate for 30 minutes, filter, wash the flask and residues with methanol in two times and transfer it to a flask, recover the solvent to dryness. Add some water to dissolving the residue, extract the aqueous solution with three 20ml of *n* – butanol saturated with water. Wash the combined butanol extracts with two 20ml quantities of water. Discard the water solution, evaporate *n* – butanol extracts to dryness, dissolve with 5ml of methanol, mix well and use it as the test solution. Weigh a quantity of saikosaponind CRS, dissolve in methanol to produce a reference solution containing 0. 2mg of saikosapponind per ml. Carry out the method for thin layer chromatography, using silica gel G as the coating substance and the lower layer of a mixture of chloroform, ethyl acetate, methanol and water (15∶40∶22∶10), standed below 10℃, as the mobile phase. Apply separately 4μl of each of the above two solutions to the plate. After developing and removal of the plate, dry in air. Spray with a 2% solution of *p* – dimethylaminobenzaldehyde in 40% sulfuric acid solution, heat at 60℃ to spots clear. Examine in daylight and under the ultraviolet light at 365nm, the yellow fluorescent spot in the chromatogram obtained with the test solution corresponds in position and colour to the spots in the chromatogram obtained with the reference solution.

2. Quantitative analysis

(1) Preparation of test solution Carry out the same method described in "Qualitative analysis".

(2) Preparation of reference solution Weigh a quantity of saikosaponin d CRS, dissolve in methanol to produce a solution containing 1mg of saikosapponin d per ml as the reference solution.

(3) Preparation of standard curve Weigh accurately 0.2ml, 0.4ml, 0.6ml, 0.8ml, 1.0ml of the above reference solution to 1ml volumetric flask, respectively, dilute with methanol to volume and mix well. Transfer accurately 0.2ml of each of solution to a 10ml stopper test tube, respectively, add 0.1ml of 1% solution of *p* – dimethylaminobenzaldehyde in ethanol, heat at 70℃ for 10 minutes, take out and cool, add 4.0ml of phosphoric acid, react for 30 minutes at 70℃, cool again. Measure the absorbance at 545nm and plot the standard curve, using the absorbance as ordinate and the quantity of saikosapponin d as abscissa, and calculate the correlation coefficient.

(4) Assay Weigh accurately 0.2ml of test solution, carry out the same method as described under "Preparation of standard curve", measure the absorbance of the test solution at 545nm, and calculate the content according to the standard curve.

Experiment records

1. Describe the process of this experiment briefly, and record the phenomena.

2. Draw the qualitative thin layer chromatogram, and calculate the R_f value of major spots.

3. Plot the standard curve and calculate the regression equation and correlation coefficient.

4. Calculate the content of Total Saikosaponins in Bupleuri Radix.

Questions

1. What other visualizing reagents can be used in quantitative analysis of saponin?

2. Please design another experimental scheme to identify Bupleuri Radix qualitatively.

Background Information

1. Origins Chinese Thorowax Root is the dried root of *Bupleurum chinense* DC. or *Bupleurum scorzonerifolium* Willd.

2. Chemical constituents Major chemical constituents of Bupleuri Radix are saponins, flavones, volatile oil, coumarins, sterols, polysaccharides and other components. Among these, saponins mainly includes saikosaponins a, b, c, d. saikosaponin d is a white powder, molecular weight is 780.98, molecular formula is $C_{42}H_{68}O_{13}$, melting point is 212 ~ 218℃, without UV absorption.

3. Actions and indications To disperse and reduce fever, soothe the liver to resolve depression, upraise *yang qi*. Common cold with fever, alternating chills and fever, distending pain in the chest and the hypochondrium, menstrual irregularities, uterine prolapsed, and prolapsed of the rectum.

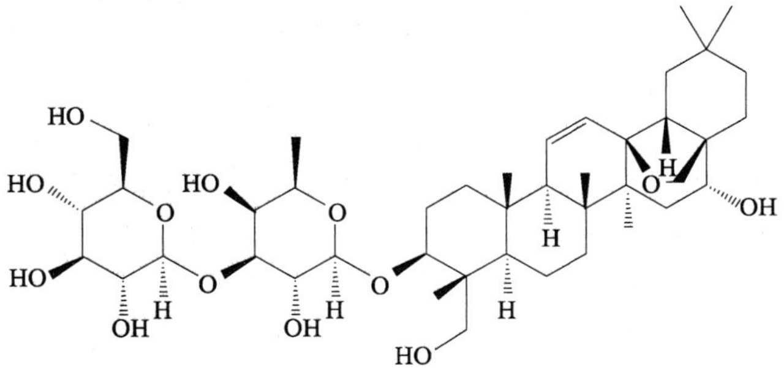

saikosaponin d

实验二　甘草中甘草酸的定性定量分析

【实验目的】

1. 掌握皂苷类成分的一般精制方法。

2. 熟悉高效液相色谱的分离原理及仪器的使用保养方法。

【实验原理】

高效液相色谱是以液体为流动相，被分离组分由于在固定相上吸附或分配不同从而使各成分得到分离。

【实验器材】

1. 仪器　高效液相色谱仪、ODS 色谱柱、电子分析天平、超声波清洗器、硅胶 G 薄层板、量瓶、三用紫外分析仪。

2. 试药与试剂　甘草饮片、甘草酸铵对照品、石油醚、甲醇、正丁醇、1% 氢氧化钠溶液、乙酸乙酯、甲酸、冰醋酸、10% 硫酸乙醇、醋酸铵。

【实验步骤】

1. 定性分析　取甘草样品粉末 1g，加石油醚 40ml，加热回流 1 小时，滤过，药渣加甲醇 30ml，加热回流 1 小时，滤过，滤液蒸干，残渣加水 40ml 使溶解，用正丁醇提取 3 次，每次 20ml，合并正丁醇液，用水洗涤 3 次，蒸干，残渣加甲醇 5ml 使溶解，作为供试品溶液。另取甘草酸铵对照品，加甲醇制成每 1ml 含 2mg 的溶液，作为对照品溶液。吸取上述溶液各 1 ~ 2μl，分别点于同一用 1% 氢氧化钠溶液制备的硅胶 G 薄层板上，以乙酸乙酯 - 甲酸 - 冰醋酸 - 水（15∶1∶1∶2）为展开剂，展开，取出，晾干，喷以 10% 的硫酸乙醇溶液，在 105℃ 加热至斑点清晰，置紫外灯（365nm）下检视。

2. 定量分析

（1）色谱条件与系统适应性试验　色谱柱为 C_{18} 柱（4.6mm × 250mm，5μm）；流动相为甲醇－0.2mol/L 醋酸铵溶液－冰醋酸（67∶32∶1）；柱温 30℃；流速 1ml/min；检测波长为 250nm。理论板数按甘草酸峰计算应不低于 3000。

（2）对照品溶液的制备　精密称取甘草酸铵盐 10mg，置 100ml 容量瓶中，甘草酸铵盐用流动相溶解，摇匀，即得。

（3）供试品溶液的制备　分别精密称取甘草饮片中粉约 0.3g，置 50ml 量瓶中，加流动相 45ml 超声处理 30 分钟，取出，放冷，加流动相至刻度，摇匀，滤过，取滤液，备用。

（4）测定法　分别精密吸取上述两种溶液适量，注入液相色谱仪，记录峰面积，计算甘草饮片中甘草酸的含量。

【实验记录】

1. 记录实验过程，绘制定性鉴别色谱图。
2. 计算甘草中甘草酸的含量。

【思考题】

1. 简述使用高效液相色谱仪的注意事项。
2. 应用 HPLC－UV 法测定皂苷类成分有何要求？

【相关资料】

1. 药材来源　本品为豆科植物甘草 *Glycyrrhiza uralensis* Fisch.、胀果甘草 *Glycyrrhiza inflate* Bat. 或光果甘草 *Glycyrrhiza glabra* L. 的干燥根及根茎。

2. 主要化学成分　甘草主要含有三萜皂苷，如甘草酸、甘草次酸等，此外，尚含黄酮类、生物碱和氨基酸等成分。甘草酸又称甘草甜素（Glycyrrhizic acid），白色或淡黄色结晶性粉末，分子式为 $C_{42}H_{62}O_{16}$，分子量 822.9，熔点 220～222℃，甘草酸具有特殊的甜味，其甜度约为蔗糖的 250 倍，溶于热水和热的稀乙醇，不溶于无水乙醇和乙醚。

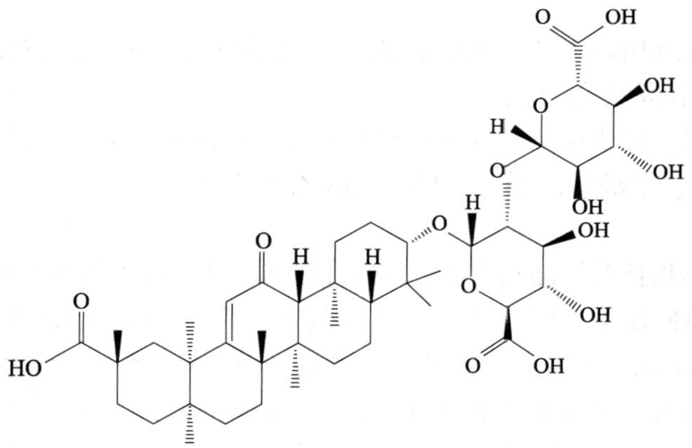

甘草酸

3. 功能与主治　甘草具有补脾益气，清热解毒，祛痰止咳，缓急止痛，调和诸药的功效。常用于脾胃虚弱，倦怠乏力，心悸气短等症。

Experiment 2 The Qualitative and Quantitative Analysis of Glycyrrhizic Acid in Glycyrrhizae Radix et Rhizoma

Purpose

1. Comprehend the general refining methods of saponin compounds.

2. Understand the separation principle of HPLC as well as the use and maintenance of the instrument.

Principle

HPLC uses a liquid as the mobile phase, and sample components can be separated due to their differences in adsorption or partition on the stationary phase.

Conditions

1. Apparatus HPLC instrument, ODS column, ultrasonic cleaner, silica gel G plate, volumetric flask and ultraviolet analyzer.

2. Reagents and materials Prepared slices of Glycyrrhiza Radix et Rhizoma, ammonium glycyrrhizinate CRS, petroleum ether, methanol, *n* – butanol, 1% NaOH, ethyl acetate, formic acid, glacial acetic acid, 10% sulfuric acid in ethanol and ammonium acetate.

Experimental Procedure

1. Qualitative analysis To 1g of the powder of Glycyrrhizae Radix et Rhizoma, add 40ml of petroleum ether, heat under reflux for 1 hour, filter and discard the ether extract. Add 30ml of methanol to the residue, heat under reflux for 1 hour and filter. Evaporate the filtrate to dryness and dissolve the residue in 40ml of water. Extract the aqueous solution with three 20ml quantities of *n* – butanol. Combine the *n* – butanol extracts, wash with water for 3 times, discard the washings, evaporate the *n* – butanol solution to dryness, and dissolve the residue in 5ml of methanol as the test solution. Dissolve a quantity of ammonium glycyrrhizinate CRS in methanol to produce a solution containing 2mg per ml as the reference solution.

Using silica gel G mixed with 1% sodium hydroxide as the coating substance and a mixture of ethyl acetate, formic acid, glacial acetic acid and water (15∶1∶1∶2) as the mobile phase. Apply separately 1 ~ 2μl of each of the two solutions to the plate. After developing and removal the plate, dry in air. Spray with 10% sulfuric acid in ethanol, heat at 105℃ to visualize clearly, and examine under the ultraviolet light at 365nm.

2. Quantitative analysis

(1) Chromatographic system and system suitability C_{18} column (4.6mm × 250mm, 5μm), mobile phase: methanol – 0.2mol/L ammonium acetate – glacial acetic acid (67∶32∶1); column temperature: 30℃, flow rate: 1ml/min; detector wavelength: 250nm. The number of the theoretical plates of the column is not less than 3000, calculated with reference to the peak of glycyrrhizic acid.

(2) Reference solution Weigh accuratately 10mg of ammonium glycyrrhizinate and

dilute with mobile phase solution to volume in a 100ml volumetric flask and mix well.

(3) Test solution Weigh accurately about 0.3g of the powder to a 50ml volumetric flask, dilute with 45ml of mobile phase solution, ultrasonicate for 30 minutes, cool and add mobile phase solution to volume. Mix well, filter and use the filtrate for testing.

(4) Procedure Accurately inject a quantity of each of the two solutions into the column separately, determine and calculate the content of glycyrrhizic acid in Glycyrrhizae Radix et Rhizoma.

Experiment records

1. Describe the process of this experiment briefly.
2. Draw thin layer chromatogram of qualitative analysis.
3. Calculate the content of glycyrrhizic acid in Glycyrrhizae Radix et Rhizoma.

Questions

1. Describe the principle precautions in the use of HPLC briefly.
2. What is the requirement to analysis saponin compounds by HPLC – UV?

Background Information

1. Origins Liquorice Root is the dried root and rhizome of *Glycyrrhiza uralensis* Fisch., *Glycyrrhiza inflate* Bat. or *Glycyrrhiza glabra* L..

2. Chemical constituents The main components of *Glycyrrhizae Radix* et Rhizoma are the triterpene saponins, such as glycyrrhizic acid and glycyrrhetinic acid. In addition, flavonoids, alkaloids and amino acids have also been mentioned. Glycyrrhetinic acid is a white or straw yellow crystalline powder, MF $C_{42}H_{62}O_{16}$, MW 822.9, mp 220 ~ 222℃, special sweet in taste, and is about 250 times sweeter than sucrose. It is soluble in hot water and diluted alcohol solution, but insoluble in absolute ethanol and ether.

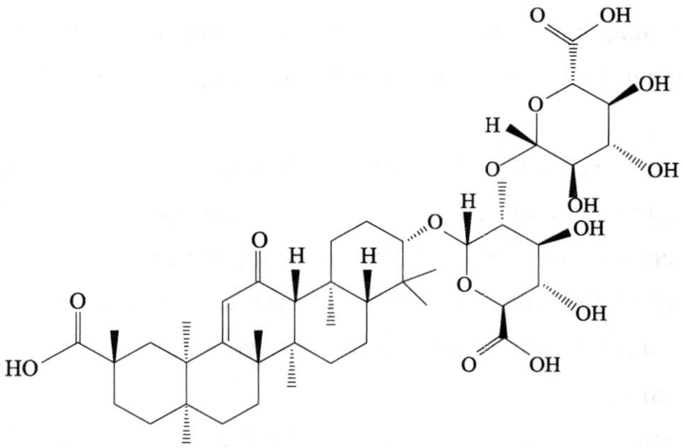

glycyrrhizic acid

3. Actions and indications Liquorice Root is to tonify spleen and tonify *qi*, clear *heat* and remove toxin, dispel phlegm to suppress cough, relax spasm and relieve pain, and moderate drug actions. And it is commonly used in spleen – stomach weakness, fatigue and lack of strength, palpitation and shortness of breath, etc..

实验三　三七中皂苷类成分的定性定量分析

【实验目的】

1. 掌握蒸发光散射检测器测定皂苷类成分的原理。

2. 熟悉皂苷类成分的主要理化性质。

【实验原理】

蒸发光散射检测器是一种通用型检测器，其响应值与被分析物质颗粒的数量和大小有关，适用于无紫外吸收或紫外吸收差的物质的检测。

【实验器材】

1. 仪器　高效液相色谱仪，蒸发光散射检测器，硅胶G薄层板，量瓶，ODS色谱柱，索氏提取器，三用紫外分析仪。

2. 试药与试剂　三七药材，三七皂苷 R_1，人参皂苷 R_{g1}，人参皂苷 R_{b1} 对照品，乙腈，三氯甲烷，正丁醇，甲醇，乙酸乙酯，10%硫酸溶液，石油醚。

【实验步骤】

1. 定性分析　取三七药材粉末1g，加三氯甲烷40ml，加热回流1小时，弃去三氯甲烷液，药渣挥干溶剂，加水0.5ml搅拌湿润，加水饱和的正丁醇10ml，超声处理30分钟，吸取上清液加3倍量氨试液，摇匀，放置分层，取上层液蒸干，残渣加甲醇1ml使溶解，作为供试品溶液。取三七皂苷 R_1、人参皂苷 R_{g1}、人参皂苷 R_{b1} 对照品适量，加甲醇制成每1ml各含1mg的混合溶液，作为对照品溶液。吸取上述两种溶液各1～5μl，分别点于同一硅胶G薄层板上，以三氯甲烷－乙酸乙酯－甲醇－水（15∶40∶22∶10）10℃以下放置的下层溶液为展开剂，展开，取出，晾干，喷以10%的硫酸溶液，在105℃加热至斑点显色清晰。供试品色谱中，在与对照品色谱相应的位置上，显相同颜色的斑点；置紫外灯下检视，显相同的荧光斑点。

2. 定量分析

（1）色谱条件　色谱柱为 C_{18} 柱（4.6mm×150mm，5μm）；流动相为乙腈－水，梯度洗脱（0min，30%乙腈～70%水，21min，60%乙腈～40%水）；流速0.6ml/min；ELSD检测器漂移管温度105℃；载气流速2.9L/min；理论板数按人参皂苷 R_{b1} 峰计算应不低于5000。

（2）供试品溶液的制备　取本品粉末（过3号筛）0.4g，精密称定，置索氏提取器中，加石油醚适量，加热回流1小时，弃去醚液，药渣挥去石油醚，置于索氏提取器中，加甲醇适量，加热提取至无色，取甲醇提取液，挥干，残渣加甲醇溶解，定量转移至25ml量瓶中，加甲醇至刻度，摇匀，作为供试品溶液。

（3）对照品溶液的制备　分别精密称取三七皂苷 R_1、人参皂苷 R_{g1}、R_{b1} 对照品适量，加甲醇制成每1ml分别含0.15、0.49、0.40mg的混合溶液，即得。

（4）样品测定　分别精密吸取对照品溶液5μl、10μl与供试品溶液10μl，注入液相色谱仪，依上述色谱条件测定，以外标两点法分别计算三七皂苷 R_1、人参皂苷 R_{g1} 和 R_{b1} 的含量。

【实验记录】

1. 记录实验过程及现象。

2. 绘制定性鉴别色谱图，计算主要斑点的 R_f 值。

3. 计算三七药材中三七皂苷 R_1、人参皂苷 R_{g1} 及 R_{b1} 的含量。

【思考题】

简述蒸发光散射检测器的工作原理和使用注意点。

【相关资料】

1. 药材来源　本品为五加科植物三七 *Panax notoginseng*（Burk.）F. H. Chen 的干燥根及根茎。

2. 主要化学成分　三七主要含有皂苷类成分，多数为达玛烷型，有三七皂苷 R_1、R_2，人参皂苷 R_{b1}、R_{b2}、R_{b3}、R_e、R_{g1}、R_{h1} 等，此外，还含有黄酮、挥发油、甾醇等成分。三七皂苷 R_1 为白色无定形粉末（甲醇），分子量为930.5，熔点215～217℃，溶于水、甲醇和乙醇，易溶于热水，不溶于乙醚、三氯甲烷和苯。人参皂苷 R_{g1} 的分子量为830.03，无色半结晶物（正丁醇－甲基乙基酮），熔点194～196.5℃，溶于甲醇、吡啶及热丙酮，稍溶于乙酸乙酯、三氯甲烷。人参皂苷 R_{b1} 为白色无定形粉末（甲醇），分子量1106.5，熔点197～198℃，溶于水、甲醇和乙醇，不溶于乙醚和苯。

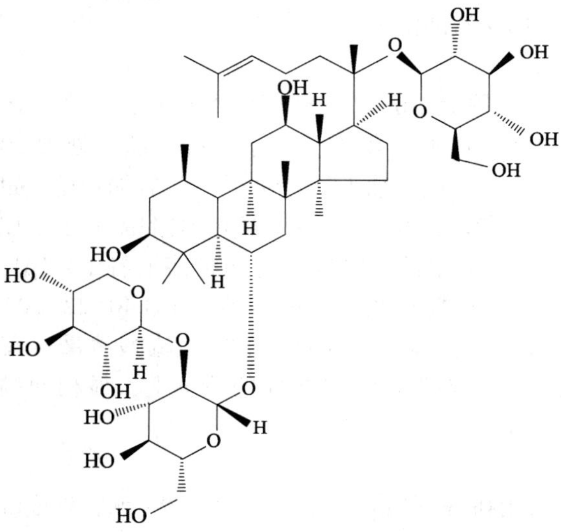

三七皂苷R_1

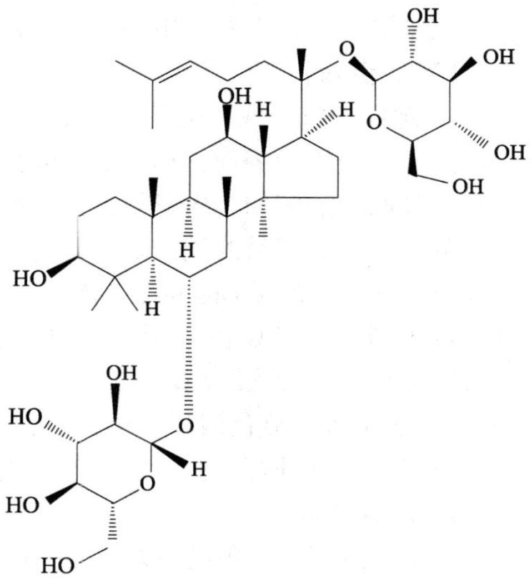

三七皂苷R_1

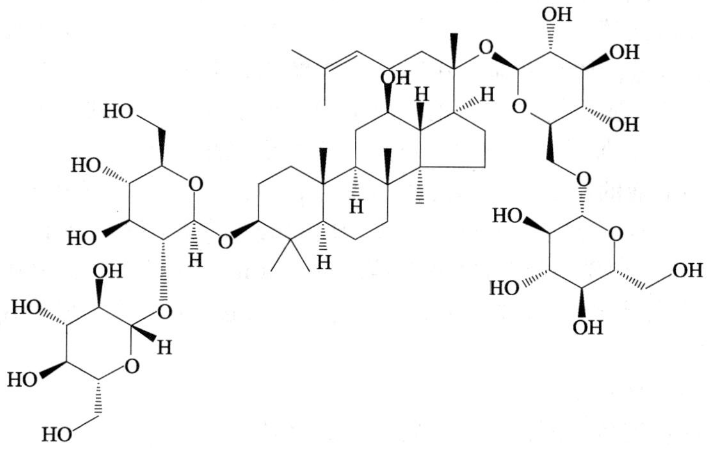

人参皂苷Rb_1

3. 功能与主治 散瘀止血，消肿定痛。用于咯血、吐血、便血、崩漏，外伤出血，胸腹刺痛，跌扑肿痛。

Experiment 3 The Qualitative and Quantitative Analysis of Saponins in Notoginseng Radix et Rhizoma

Purpose

1. Comprehend the principle of evaporative light scattering detector in determination of saponins.

2. Understand the main physical and chemical properties of saponins.

Principle

Evaporative light scattering detector is a kind of universal detector whose response value is concerned with the quantity and size of material particles to be analyzed. It is employed in detection of substances with no or lower ultraviolet absorption.

Conditions

1. Apparatus HPLC instrument, evaporative light scattering detector, silica gel G plate, volumetric flask, ODS column, Soxhlet's extractor, ultraviolet analyzer.

2. Reagents and materials Notoginseng Radix et Rhizoma, Notoginsenoside R_1、ginsenoside R_{g_1} and R_{b_1} CRS, acetonitrile, chloroform, *n* – butanol, methanol, ethyl acetate, 10% sulfuric acid solution and petroleum ether.

Experimental Procedure

1. Qualitative analysis To 1g of the powder, add 40ml of chloroform, heat under reflux on a water bath for 1 hour, discard the chloroform extract, evaporate the residue to dryness, misten the residue with 0.5ml of water, add 10ml of *n* – butanol saturated with water, ultrasonicate for 30 minutes. To the supernatant liquid add 3 volumes of ammonia TS, mix well, stand for separating. Evaporate the supernatant to dryness, dissolve the residue in 1ml of methanol as the test solution. Dissolve ginsenoside R_{b_1} CRS, notoginsenoside R_1 CRS and finsenoside R_{g_1} CRS in methanol to produce a mixture containing 1mg of each per ml as the reference solution. Apply separately to the plate 1 ~ 5μl of each of the two solutions. Carry out the method for thin layer chromatography, using silica gel G as the coating substance and the lower layer of a mixture of chloroform, ethyl acetate, methanol and water (15∶40∶22∶10), standed below 10℃ as the mobile phase. After developing and removal of the plate, dry in air. Spray with a 10% solution of sulfuric acid in ethanol and heat at 105℃ to the spots clear. The spots in the chromatogram obtained with the test solution correspond in position and colour to the spots in the chromatogram obtained with the reference solution. Or examine under ultraviolet light at 365nm, both chromatogram show the same fluorescent spots.

2. Quantitative Analysis

(1) Chromatographic system andsystem suitability Use C_{18} column (4.6mm × 150mm, 5μm); acetonitrile – water as the mobile phase, Gradient elution (0min, 30% ace-

tonitrile to 70% water, 21min, 60% acetonitrile and 40% water); flow rate: 0.6ml/min; As detector an evaporative light scattering detector is employed. Drift tube temperature: 105℃; Flow rate of carrier gas: 2.9L/min; the number of theoretical plates of the column is not less than 5000, with the reference to the peak of ginsenosides R_{b_1}.

(2) Test solution Weigh accurately 0.4g of the powder (through No. 3 sieve) to a Soxhlet's extractor, add the a quantity of petroleum ether and heated under reflux for 1 hour, discard the ether extract, expel the solvent from the residue, place in a Soxhlet's extractor, add a quantity of methanol and heated to methanol extract colorless, evaporate the methanol extract to dryness, dissolved the residue in methanol, transferr accurately to a 25ml volumetric flask, add methanol to volume and mix well as the test solution.

(3) Reference solution Dissolve ginsenoside R_{b_1} CRS, notoginsenoside R_1 CRS and ginsenoside R_{g_1} CRS, accurately weighed, to produce a mixture containing 0.15mg, 0.49mg, 0.40mg of each per ml, as the reference solution.

(4) Procedure Inject accurately 5μl, 10μl of the reference solutions and 10μl of the test solution, respectively, into the column, determine and calculate the content of Notoginsenoside R_1, ginsenosides R_{g1} and R_{b1} in sample using a calibration equation of logarithm alteration of two external standards.

Experimental Records

1. Record the experimental process and phenomena.

2. Draw chromatogram about qualitative identification and calculate R_f value of the main point.

3. Calculate the content of Notoginsenoside R_1, Ginsenoside R_{g_1} and Ginsenoside R_{b_1} in Notoginseng Radix et Rhizoma.

Questions

Describe the principle and using notices of the evaporative light scattering detector briefly.

Background Information

1. Origins Sanchi is the dried root of *Panax notoginseng* (Burk.) F. H. Chen (Fam. Araliaceae).

2. Chemical constituents Sanchi mainly contains saponins, and most are of the dammarane type, including notoginsenoside R_1, R_2, ginsenosides R_{b1}, R_{b2}, R_{b3}, R_e, R_{g1}, R_{h1}. Moreover, it also contains flavonoids, volatile oil, phytosterol and other compositions. Notoginsenoside R_1 is white amorphous powder (methanol). The molecular weight is 930.5. Melting point is 215 ~ 217℃. It is soluble in water, methanol and ethanol, easily soluble in hot water, insoluble in ethyl ether, chloroform and benzene. Ginsenosides R_{g_1} is colorless semi crystal (Butanol – methyl ethyl ketone). The molecular weight is 830.3. Melting point is 194 ~ 196.5℃. It is soluble in methanol, pyridine and hot acetone, slightly soluble in ethyl acetate、chloroform. Ginsenosides R_{b_1} is a white amorphous powder (methanol). The molecular weight is 1106.5. Melting point is 197 ~ 198℃. It is easily soluble in water, methanol and ethanol, insoluble in ethyl ether, benzene.

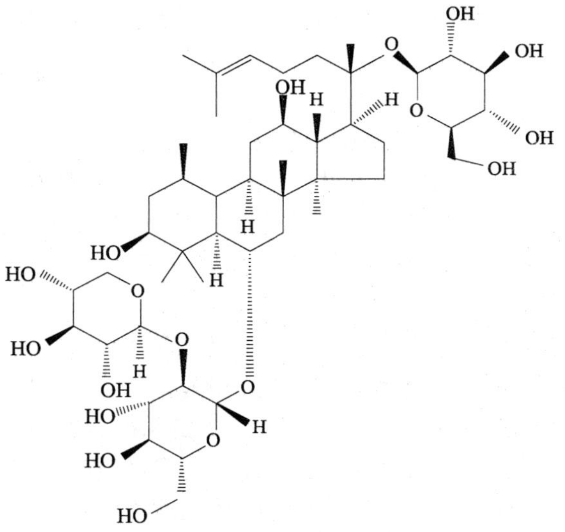

notoginsenoside R_1

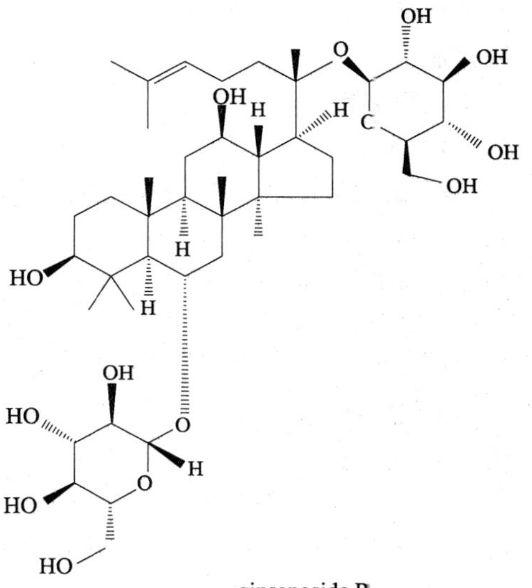

ginsenoside R_{g1}

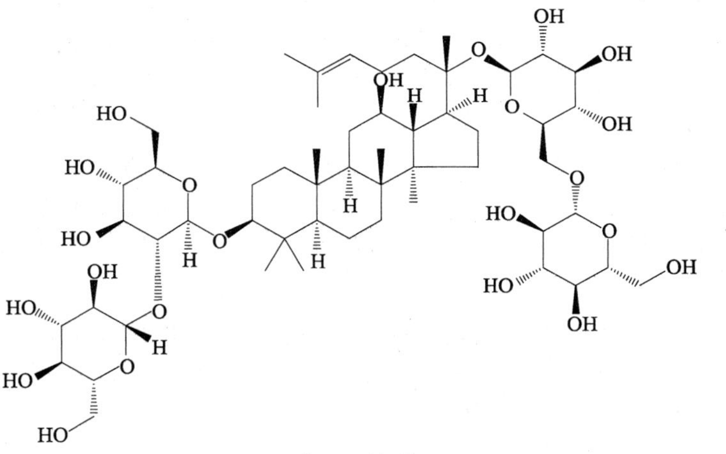

ginsenoside R_{b1}

3. Actions and indications To dissipate stasis and stanch bleeding, disperse swelling and relieve pain. Hemoptysis, hematemesis, epistaxis, hematochezia, flooding and spotting, traumatic bleeding, stabbing pain in chest and abdomen, swelling and pain caused by injuries from falls.

实验四　玉屏风口服液的定性定量分析

【实验目的】

1. 熟悉中药制剂的质量分析特点。
2. 了解中药制剂分析的一般样品处理方法。

【实验原理】

玉屏风口服液主要由黄芪、防风、白术三味药材组成，其中黄芪为主药，其主要有效成分为黄芪甲苷，本实验通过对玉屏风口服液中黄芪甲苷的定性、定量分析来控制该制剂的质量。

【实验器材】

1. 仪器 高效液相色谱仪、蒸发光散射检测器、硅胶 G 薄层板。

2. 试剂与试药 黄芪甲苷对照品，黄芪、防风、白术对照药材，玉屏风口服液、阴性样液（按处方药味除去被测药材，其余药味按制剂的制备工艺制得）。乙腈为色谱纯、水为重蒸馏水、正丁醇、40%氨水、10%硫酸乙醇。

【实验步骤】

1. 定性分析 取本品 10ml 以水饱和的正丁醇萃取 3 次，每次 10ml，合并正丁醇液以 40%氨水 30ml 洗涤 1 次，弃去碱水层，将正丁醇层蒸干，残渣加甲醇 1ml 溶解，作为供试品溶液。另取黄芪对照药材 5g 加水煎煮 1.5 小时，滤过，滤液加乙醇使含醇量达 60%，静置，滤过，滤液蒸干，残渣加水溶解后按供试品溶液制备方法制成对照药材溶液。另取黄芪甲苷对照品，加甲醇制成每 1ml 含 1mg 的溶液，作为对照品溶液。取缺黄芪的阴性样液按供试品溶液的制备方法制成阴性对照溶液。吸取上述 4 种溶液各 4～6μl，分别点于同一硅胶 G 薄层板上，以三氯甲烷－甲醇－水（65∶35∶10）下层为展开剂，展开，取出，晾干，喷以 10%的硫酸乙醇溶液，在 105℃烘约 5 分钟，供试品色谱中，在与对照药材和对照品色谱相应的位置上，显相同的紫红色斑点，阴性对照液色谱无干扰。

2. 定量分析

（1）色谱条件 色谱柱为 C_{18}（250mm×4.6mm）柱；流动相：乙腈－水（37∶63）；流速：0.8ml/min；进样量：20μl；ELSD 参数：漂移管温度为 100℃，氮气流速为 2.2L/min。

（2）对照品溶液的配制 精密称取黄芪甲苷对照品适量，以甲醇溶解并定容，配成 1mg/ml 的溶液。

（3）供试品溶液的制备 精密吸取本品 5ml，以水饱和的正丁醇 5ml 萃取 6 次，合并正丁醇液，以 40%氨水 25ml 洗涤。弃去碱水层，将正丁醇层回收至干，用甲醇溶解并定容至 10ml，测定时过微孔滤膜。

（4）测定法 分别精密吸取上述两种溶液 20μl 进样，记录峰面积，计算玉屏风口服液中黄芪甲苷的含量。

【实验记录】

1. 记录实验过程，绘制定性鉴别色谱图。

2. 计算玉屏风口服液中黄芪甲苷的含量。

【思考题】

简述中药制剂定性鉴别实验的注意点。

【相关资料】

1. 药材来源 本品为中药黄芪、防风和白术制成的口服液，是中医扶正固表的传统名方。

2. 主要化学成分 玉屏风口服液由黄芪、防风和白术组成，黄芪主要含有黄芪皂苷、异黄芪皂苷、大豆皂苷等皂苷类成分，其中黄芪甲苷是主要有效成分之一。此外，还含有黄芪多糖、黄酮类成分等。防风主要含有升麻苷、升麻素、5－O－甲基维斯阿米醇苷等。白术含有白术内酯、苍术酮、倍半萜类、多炔醇类等成分。黄芪甲苷为白色无定形粉末，分子量784.97分子式$C_{41}H_{68}O_{14}$，熔点299～300℃（甲醇）。

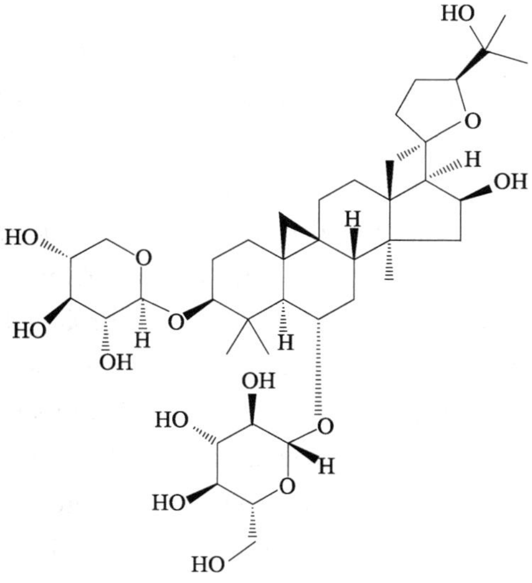

黄芪甲苷

3. 功能与主治　具有益气、固表、止汗作用，用于表虚不固，自汗恶风，面色㿠白，或体虚易感风邪者。

（夏玉凤）

Experiment 4　The Qualitative and Quantitative Analysis of Yupingfeng Mixture

Purpose

1. Understand the characteristics of quality analysis of chinese medicine preparation.

2. Know about the general processing method of analysis of Chinese medicine preparation.

Principle

Yupingfeng Mixture is composed of astragalus mongholicus, saposhnikovia divaricata and rhizoma atractylodis macrocephalae. Astragalus mongholicus is the monarch drug in the prescription, with the main effective ingredient is astragaloside Ⅳ. In this experiment, we control the quality of the preparation of Yupingfeng kufuye through the qualitative and quantitative analysis of astragaloside Ⅳ.

Conditions

1. Apparatus　HPLC instrument and evaporative light scattering detector.

2. Reagents and materials　Astragaloside Ⅳ CRS, Astragali Radix reference drug, Saposhnikoviae Radix reference drug, Atractylodis Macrocephalae Rhizoma, Yupingfeng Mixture, negative sample solution, acetonitrile (chromatographic pure), double distilled water, *n* –

butanol, 40% ammonia water and 10% sulphuric acid in ethanol.

Experimental Procedure

1. Qualitative analysis Extract 10ml by shaking with three 10ml quantities of *n* – butanol saturated with water. Combine the *n* – butanol extracts, wash with 30ml of 40% ammonia water. Evaporate the *n* – butanol extracts to dryness, and dissolve the residue in 1ml of methanol as the test solution. Take 5g stragalus reference drug, decocted with water for 1.5 hour, filter, add alcohol until the content of alcohol is 60%, stand and filter. Evaporate the filtrate to dryness and dissolve the residue in water to prepare the reference drug solution as the same method described as the test solution. Dissolve a quantity of astragaloside Ⅳ CRS in methanol to procedure a solution containing 1mg per ml as the reference solution. Prepare the negative control solution by taking the negative sample solution without radix astragali according to the preparation of test solution. Carry out the method for thin layer chromatography, using silica gel G as the coating substance and the lower layer of a mixture of chloroform, methanol and water (65∶35∶10) as the mobile phase. Apply separately 4 ~ 6μl of each of the four solutions to the plate. After developing and removal of the plate, dry in air, spray with 10% sulphuric acid in ethanol and heat at 105℃ for 5min to the spots clear. The spot in the chromatogram obtained with the test solution corresponds in position and colour to the spot in the chromatogram obtained with the reference solution. There is no interference in the chromatogram of negative reference solution.

2. Quantitative analysis

(1) Chromatographic system and system suitability C_{18} column (250mm × 4.6mm); a mixture of acetonitrile and water (37∶63) as the mobile phase; flow rate: 0.8ml/min; volume of sample: 20μl; ELSD parameter: drift tube temperature 100℃; Nitrogen flow rate: 2.2L/min.

(2) Reference solution Dissolve a quantity of astragaloside Ⅳ CRS, weighed accurately, in methanol to prepare a solution containing 1mg per ml.

(3) Test solution Extract 5ml of the mixture, measured accurately, with six 5ml quantities of *n* – butanol saturated with water, combine the extract, and wash with 25ml quantities of 40 % ammonia water. Recover and evaporate the solvent to dryness, dissolve the residue in methanol to a 10ml volumetric flask. All above solutions should filter through the microporous membrane before injection.

(4) Procedure Inject accurately 20μl of each of the above solution into the column, respectively. Determine and calculate the content of astragaloside Ⅳ in Yupingfeng Mixture.

Experimental Records

1. Describe the experiment procedure.
2. Draw the qualitative chromatogram.
3. Calculate the content of astragaloside Ⅳ in Yupingfeng Mixture.

Questions

Which procedure should be paid more attention to in the qualitative analysis?

Background Information

1. Origins　Yupingfeng Mixture is the oral liquid composed of astragalus mongholicus, saposhnikovia divaricata and rhizoma atractylodis macrocephalae, and it is a classical prescription of strengthen the superficies.

2. Chemical constituents　Yupingfeng Mixture is composed of Astragali Radix, Saposhnikoviae Radix and Atractylodis Macrocephalae Rhizoma. Astragali Radix mainly contains astragalosides, isoastragalosides and soyasaponins, with astragaloside Ⅳ is one of the main effective components. Furthermore, it contains astragalus polysaccharides and flavonoids. Saposhnikovia divaricata mainly contains prim – *O* – glucosylcimifugin, cimifugin and 4′ – *O* – *β* – Glucopyranosyl – 5 – *O* – Methylvisamminol. Atractylodis Macrocephalae Rhizoma contains atractylenolide – 1, atractyloxide, sesquiterpenes, multi propargyl alcohol and so on. Astragaloside Ⅳ is a white amorphous powder and the molecular weight is 784. 97, molecular formula: $C_{41}H_{68}O_{14}$; Melting point: 299 ~ 300℃ (CH_3OH).

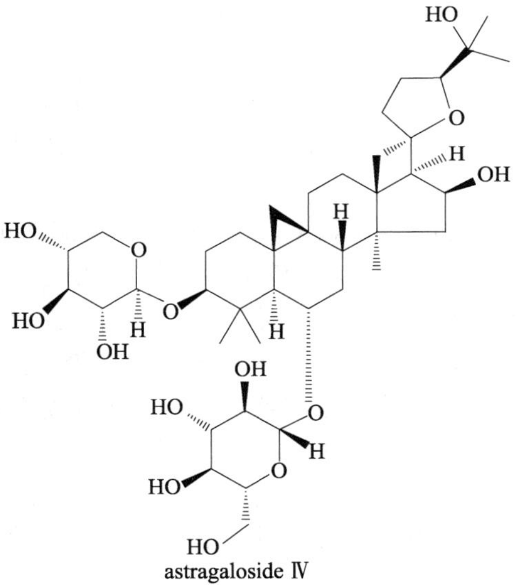

astragaloside Ⅳ

3. Actions and indications　Spontaneous sweating and aversion to wind, and pallar due to exterior deficiency, or weak patients who are susceptible to wind.

(Yufeng Xia)

第五章
挥发油类成分的分析

实验一　薄荷素油的定性定量分析

【实验目的】

1. 掌握薄荷素油中主要单萜类活性成分的定性定量分析方法。

2. 熟悉气相色谱法在中药挥发性成分分析中的应用和特点。

【实验原理】

气相色谱法（Gas Chromatography，GC）是以气体为流动相的色谱方法。气相色谱的过程是将要分离的样品（组分）由一种惰性气体（载气）携带通过层析柱（色谱柱），样品中的混合组分在载气和固定液之间分配，固定液根据样品的分配系数，有选择地对它们加以阻滞，直到它们在载气中形成分离的谱带为止。这些谱带随载气流出色谱柱，并按先后次序经过检测器，检测器将载气中各组分的浓度变化转变为相应的电讯号，作为时间函数，由记录仪以峰的形式记录下来，即为色谱图。

薄荷素油为无色或淡黄色液体，含多种挥发性成分，如薄荷脑，薄荷酮，乙酸薄荷酯等。由于薄荷脑是薄荷油中的主要活性成分且其含量较高，因此是对薄荷素油进行质量控制的主要指标性成分。

聚乙二醇类是气相色谱柱中常用的极性固定相，依据相似相溶原理，此类色谱柱常用于极性成分的分析。薄荷脑为环醇结构，沸点在200℃以上。本实验以改性聚乙二醇作为固定相，可不同程度地吸附中等或小极性成分。通过程序升温法将薄荷脑和其他不同沸点的挥发性成分分离开来。

【实验器材】

1. 仪器　气相色谱仪、氢火焰离子化检测器、DB - WAX 聚乙二醇（PEG）气相毛细管柱、微量进样器、展开缸等。

2. 试药与试剂　薄荷素油、薄荷脑对照品、无水乙醇、硅胶 GF_{254} 薄层板、甲苯 - 乙酸乙酯（19:1）、茴香醛试液。

3. 内标物　萘。

【实验步骤】

1. 定性分析　取本品 0.1g，加无水乙醇 5ml 使溶解，作为供试品溶液。另取薄荷素油对照提取物，同法制成对照提取物溶液。照薄层色谱法试验，吸取上述两种溶液各5μl，分别点于同一硅胶 GF_{254} 薄层板上，以甲苯 - 乙酸乙酯（19∶1）为展开剂，展开，取出，晾干，置紫外光灯（254nm）下检视。供试品色谱中，在与对照提取物色谱相应的位置上，显相同颜色的斑点。喷以茴香醛试液，在105℃加热至斑点显色清晰。供试品色谱中，在与对照提取物色谱相应的位置上，显相同颜色的斑点；置紫外光灯（365nm）下检视，显相同颜色的荧光斑点。

2. 定量分析

（1）色谱条件与系统适用性试验　以改性聚乙二醇为固定相的毛细管柱（柱长为30m，内径为0.25mm，膜厚度为0.25μm）；程序升温：初始温度60℃，保持4分钟，以每分钟2℃的速率升温至100℃，再以每分钟10℃的速率升温至230℃，保持1分钟；进样口温度250℃；检测器温度：250℃；分流进样，分流比5∶1。理论板数按萘峰计算应不低于20000。

（2）校正因子测定　取萘适量，精密称定，加无水乙醇制成每1ml含1.8mg的溶液，摇匀，作为内标溶液。另取薄荷脑对照品约30mg，精密称定，置10ml量瓶中，加内标溶液至刻度，摇匀，吸取1μl注入气相色谱仪，计算校正因子。

（3）测定法　取本品约80mg，精密称定，置10ml量瓶中，加内标溶液至刻度，摇匀，吸取1μl注入气相色谱仪，测定，即得。

【实验记录】

1. 绘制定性薄层色谱图，记录薄荷油中主要斑点的 R_f 值及颜色。

2. 根据气相色谱法结果，采用内标法计算薄荷素油中薄荷脑的含量。

【思考题】

1. 气相色谱法中，样品含量的计算有面积归一化法，峰高法，外标法和内标法，请问不同的计算方法各有什么特点？

2. 实验过程中载气流量的变化对定量分析结果会有何影响？

3. 除聚乙二醇为固定相的毛细管柱可以用于薄荷中薄荷脑的分析外，还有哪些系列的毛细管柱也可应用于薄荷脑的分析？

【相关资料】

1. 来源　本品为唇形科植物薄荷 *Mentha haplocalyx* Briq. 的新鲜茎和叶经水蒸气蒸馏、冷冻、部分脱脑加工提取的挥发油。

2. 薄荷素油中的化学成分　薄荷素油中主要含 *l* - 薄荷脑77% ~87%，*l* - 薄荷酮约10%，乙酸薄荷酯1% ~6%。薄荷素油质量的优劣主要依据其中薄荷脑含量的高低而定。

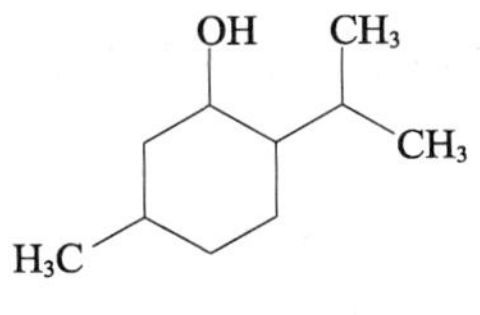

薄荷脑

3. 功能与主治　薄荷：疏散风热，清利头目，利咽，透疹，疏肝行气。用于风热感冒，风温初起，头痛，目赤，喉痹，口疮，风疹，麻疹，胸胁胀闷。

Experiment 1 The Qualitative and Quantitative Analysis of Peppermint Oil

Purpose

1. Comprehend the qualitative and quantitative analysis of the main active ingredient of monoterpenoids in peppermint oil.

2. Understand applications and features of gas chromatography in analysis of volatile components in traditional Chinese medicines.

Principle

Gas chromatography (GC) is a separation technique in which the carrier gas is passing through the chromatographic column packed with stationary liquid for separation and determination. The substances are injected to the vaporizer with a microsyringe and vaporized, separated on the stationary phase, each component passes through the detector in succession and a chromatogram is thus recorded by integrator, recorder or data acquisition system.

Peppermint oil is a colorless or pale yellow liquid contained with many volatile components, e. g. *l* - menthol, *l* - menthone and menthyl acetate. Menthol is the main chemical marker for the quality control because of its activity and high content.

Polyethylene glycol is commonly used as polar stationary phase in GC. Basing on the theory of "similarity and intermiscibility", this kind of column is usually used in separation of polar compounds. Menthol has the cyclitol structure and the boiling point of this compound is above 200℃. In this experiment, modified polyethylene glycol is used as the stationary phase to separate the components with different polarities in peppermint oil. Menthol and other components can be successfully separated by the programmed temperature method.

Conditions

1. Apparatus Gas chromatograph, flame ionization detector, DB - WAX PEG capillary column, mycrosyringe and developing chamber.

2. Reagents and materials Peppermint oil, menthol reference substance, dehydrated ethanol, GF_{254} thin layer plate, methylbenzene, ethyl acetate , anisaldehyde test solution.

3. The internal standard substance Naphthalene.

Experimental Procedure

1. Qualitative analysis Dissolve 0. 1g of the volatile oil in 5ml of dehydrated ethanol as the test solution. Prepare a solution of Peppermint oil reference extract in the same manner as the reference extract solution. Carry out the method for thin layer chromatography, using silica gel GF_{254} as the coating substance and a mixture of toluene and ethyl acetate (19:1) as the mobile phase. Apply separately to the plate 5μl of each of the above two solutions. After developing and removal of the plate, dry in air. Examine under ultraviolet light at 254nm, the fluorescent spots in the chromatogram obtained with the test solution correspond in position and colour to the spots in the chromatogram obtained with the reference extract solution. Spray with anisaldehyde TS and heat at 105℃ to the spots clear. Examine in daylight, the spots in the chromatogram obtained with the test solution correspond in position and colour to the spots in the chromatogram obtained with the reference extract solution. Examine under ultraviolet light at 365nm, the fluorescent spots in the chromatogram obtained with the test solution correspond in position and colour to the spots in the chromatogram obtained with the reference extract solution.

2. Quantitative analysis

(1) Chromatographic system and system suitability　Use modified polyethylene glycol as the stationary phase (30m in length, 0.25mm in inner diameter, 0.25μm in film thickness). Programmed temperature: initial temperature at 60℃, maintain 4 minutes, increase at 2℃ per minute to 100℃, then increase at 10℃ per minute to 230℃, maintain 1 minute. The injector temperature is set at 250℃ and the detector temperature is set at 250℃. The split ratio is 5∶1. The number of theoretical plates of the column is not less than 20000, calculated with the reference to the peak of naphthalene.

(2) Correction factor　Dissolve a quantity of naphthalene, accurately weighed, in dehydrated ethanol to produce a solution containing 1.8mg per ml, mix well, as the internal standard solution. Dissolve 30mg menthol CRS, accurately weighed, in a 10ml volumetric flask and dilute with the internal standard solution to volume, and mix well. Inject accurately 1μl of the test solution into the column, and calculate the correction factor for menthol.

(3) Procedure　Dissolve about 80mg, accurately weighed, in a 10ml volumetric flask, add the internal standard solution to volume, and mix well. Inject accurately 1μl of the test solution into the column and calculate the content.

Experimental Records

1. Draw the qualitative TLC chromatogram. Record the R_f values and color of the main spots in peppermint oil.

2. According to the results of GC, calculate the content of menthol in peppermint oil with internal standard method.

Questions

1. In GC, sample content is often calculated with area normalization method, the peak height method, internal standard method or external standard method, what is the characteristic of different calculation methods?

2. During the experiment, changes in carrier gas flow rate in the process of the assay will have any effect on the results?

3. What series of capillary column can be used for the analysis of menthol except for the

capillary column with polyethylene glycol as the stationary phase?

Background Information

1. Origins Peppermint Oil is the volatile oil obtained by steam distillating, freezing, removing partly from menthol from fresh Menthae Haplocalyx Herba.

2. Chemical constituents Peppermint oil mainly contains *l* – menthol (77% ~87%), *l* – menthone (10%) and menthyl acetate (1% ~6%). Its quality bases primarily on the content of *l* – menthol.

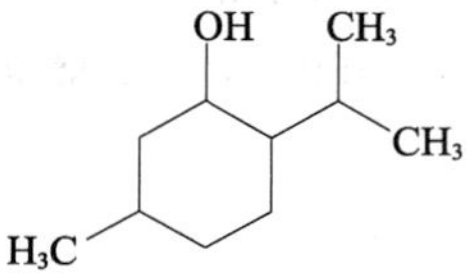

menthol

3. Actions and indications Menthae Haplocalyx Herba: To disperse wind – heat, clear and sooth head and eyes, soothe the throat, promote eruption, soothe the liver to move *qi*. Used for common cold caused by wind – heat, early onset of wind – warmth disease, headache, red eyes, throat impediment, mouth sore, rubella, measles, distention and oppression in the chest and the hypochondrium.

实验二 丁香中丁香酚的定性定量分析

【实验目的】

1. 掌握气相色谱法的操作技术。
2. 掌握丁香中挥发性活性成分的定性定量分析方法。

【实验原理】

丁香中含有挥发油高达14% ~21%，丁香酚是其中的主要成分，具有广泛的药理作用，如抗炎、抗过敏、解热、麻醉等。2015 版《中国药典》一部将丁香酚作为指标性成分，规定丁香中含有丁香酚不得少于11%。目前常用 HPLC 和 GC 两种方法对丁香酚进行定量测定。HPLC 法可对丁香中的多种化学成分进行分析，GC 法主要针对丁香中包括丁香酚在内的挥发性成分进行分析。本实验采用聚乙二醇涂布的毛细管柱分析测定丁香中丁香酚的含量。

【实验器材】

1. 仪器 气相色谱仪、氢火焰离子化检测器、DB – WAX 聚乙二醇（PEG）气相毛细管柱、微量进样器、展开缸等。

2. 试药与试剂 丁香，丁香酚对照品，乙醚，硅胶 G 薄层板，石油醚（60 ~90℃）– 乙酸乙酯（9:1），5%香草醛硫酸溶液。

【实验步骤】

1. 定性分析 取本品粉末 0.5g，加乙醚 5ml，振摇数分钟，滤过，滤液作为供试品溶液。另取丁香酚对照品，加乙醚制成每 1ml 含 16μg 的溶液，作为对照品溶液。照薄层色谱法试验，吸取上述两种溶液各 5μl，分别点于同一硅胶 G 薄层板上，以石油醚（60～90℃）－乙酸乙酯（9∶1）为展开剂，展开，取出，晾干，喷以 5% 香草醛硫酸溶液，在 105℃加热至斑点显色清晰。供试品色谱中，在与对照品色谱相应的位置上，显相同颜色的斑点。

2. 定量分析

（1）色谱条件与系统适用性试验　以聚乙二醇 20000（PEG－20M）为固定相，涂布浓度为 10%；柱温 190℃。理论板数按丁香酚峰计算应不低于 1500。

（2）对照品溶液的制备及标准曲线的绘制　精密称取丁香酚对照品 25mg，置 25ml 量瓶中，加正己烷溶解并稀释至刻度，摇匀，即得丁香酚对照品溶液（1mg/ml）。精密量取丁香酚对照品溶液 0.25、0.5、1.0、2.0、3.0、5.0ml 于 6 个 10ml 容量瓶中，用正己烷稀释、定容至刻度，混匀，各浓度进样 1μl，以峰面积为纵坐标，进样量为横坐标绘制标准曲线。

（3）供试品溶液的制备　取本品粉末（过三号筛）约 0.2g，精密称定，精密加入正己烷 20ml，称定重量，超声处理 15 分钟，放冷至室温，再称定重量，用正己烷补足减失的重量，摇匀，滤过，取续滤液，即得。

（4）测定法　精密吸取供试品溶液 1μl，注入气相色谱仪，由标准曲线计算含量。

【实验记录】

1. 绘制定性薄层图，记录丁香中主要斑点的 R_f 值及颜色。

2. 计算丁香药材中丁香酚的含量。

【思考题】

1. 目前文献中丁香酚含量测定方法常用 HPLC 和 GC 两种方法，比较两种方法的优缺点？

2. 供试品溶液制备过程中需要加正己烷补足减失的重量，有何意义？

【相关资料】

1. 药材来源　本品为桃金娘科植物丁香 *Eugenia caryophyllata* Thunb. 的干燥花蕾。当花蕾由绿色转红时采摘，晒干。

2. 丁香中的主要化学成分　花蕾含挥发油即丁香油。油中主要含有丁香酚、乙酰丁香酚、*b*－石竹烯，以及甲基正戊基酮、水杨酸甲酯、葎草烯、胡椒酚、*a*－衣兰烯等。

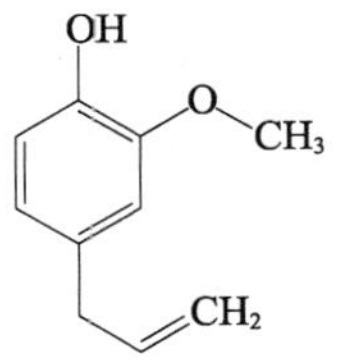

丁香酚

3. 功能与主治　温中降逆，补肾助阳。用于脾胃虚寒，呃逆呕吐，食少吐泻，心腹冷痛，肾虚阳痿。

Experiment 2 The Quantitative and Qualitative Analysis of Eugenol in Caryophylli Flos

Purpose

1. Comprehend the operation of the gas chromatography (GC) method.

2. Comprehend the qualitative and quantitative analysis method of the volatile active ingredients in Caryophylli Flos.

Principle

Caryophylli Flos contains 14% ~21% of volatile oil, eugenol is the main component. It has multiple actions, such as anti - inflammatory, anti - allergic, antipyretic and anesthesia. Eugenolis is used as the chemical marker in quality control of this drug. According to the Chinese Pharmacopoeia (2015 edition, Part One), the content of eugenolis in Caryophylli Flos should not be less than 11%. Both of HPLC and GC can be used in eugenol quantitative analysis. HPLC can be used for the assay of more components in Caryophylli Flos, while GC is mainly used for the volatile constituents concluding eugenol. Capillary column with polyethylene glycol as stationary phase is employed in this experiment for the determination of eugenol in Caryophylli Flos.

Conditions

1. Apparatus Gas chromatograph, flame ionization detector, DB - WAX PEG capillary column and mycrosyringe.

2. Reagents and materials Crude drugs of Caryophylli Flos (through No. 2 sieve), eugenol CRS, ether, silica gel G plate, petroleum ether (60 ~ 90℃), ethyl acetate and 5% solution of vanillin in sulfuric acid.

Experimental Procedure

1. Qualitative analysis To 0.5g of the powder (through No. 3 sieve), add 5ml of ether, shake for several minutes, filter and use the filtrate as the test solution. Dissolve a quantity of eugenol CRS in ether to produce a solution containing 16μg per ml as the reference solution. Carry out the method for thin layer chromatography, using silica gel G as the coating substance and a mixture of petroleum ether (60 ~90℃) and ethyl acetate (9∶1) as the mobile phase. Apply 5μl of each of the two solutions to the plate. After developing and removal of the plate, dry in air, spray with a 5% solution of vanillin in sulfuric acid and heat at 105℃ to the spots clear. The spot in the chromatogram obtained with the test solution corresponds in position and colour to the spot obtained with the reference solution.

2. Quantitative analysis

(1) Chromatographic system and system suitability Use 10% polyethylene glycol (PEG) -20M as the stationary phase and maintain the column temperature at 190℃. The number of theoretical plates of the column is not less than 1500, calculated with reference to the peak of eugenol.

(2) Reference solution and standard curve　Weigh accurately eugenol CRS 25mg to a 25ml volumetric flask, dissolve with a quantity of n – hexane and dilute to volume to prepare a solution containing 1.0mg per ml as the reference solution. Measure accurately 0.25ml, 0.5ml, 1.0ml, 2.0ml, 3.0ml, 5.0ml of the above reference solution to a 10ml volumetric flask, respectively, and add n – hexane to volume, mix well. Inject 1μl of each of the solution, respectively, into the column, plot the standard curve, using peak area as the ordinate and the content as the abscissa.

(3) Test solution　To about 0.2g of the powder, accurately weighed, add accurately 20ml of n – hexane and weigh, ultrasonicate for 15 minutes, cool to room temperature and weigh again, replenish the loss of the solvent with n – hexane, mix well and filter, use the filtrate as the test solution.

(4) Procedure　Inject accurately 1μl of the test solution into the column, determine and calculate the content by the standard curve.

Experimental Records

1. Draw the qualitative TLC chromatogram. Record the R_f values and colors of the main spots in sample chromatogram.

2. Calculate the content of eugenol in Caryophylli Flos.

Questions

1. HPLC and GC are commonly used for the quantitative analysis of eugenol. What are the advantages and disadvantages of two methods?

2. The process of test solution preparation requires adding n – hexane to replenish the weight loss, what is the purpose of this procedure?

Background Information

1. Origins　Caryophylli Flos is the dried flower bud of *Eugenia caryophyllata* Thunb. (Fam. Myrtaceae). The drug is collected when it turns from green to brick – red, and dried in the sun.

2. Chemical constituents　Flower buds contain volatile oil namely clove oil. It mainly concludes eugenol, acetyl – eugenol, b – caryophyllene, methyl – n – amyl ketone, methyl salicylate, humuleno, chavicol and a – ylangene etc..

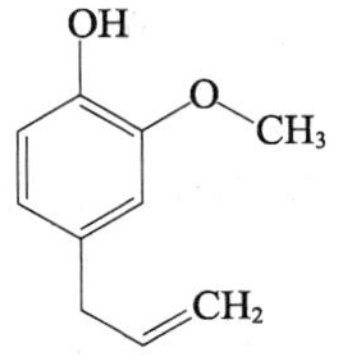

eugenol

3. Actions and indications　To warm the middle energizer and downbear counterflow, tonify the kidney and assist yang. Used for spleen – stomach deficiency cold; hiccup and vomiting; low appetite, vomiting and diarrhea; cold pain in the heart and abdomen, impotence caused by kidney deficiency.

实验三　莪术油的定性定量分析

【实验目的】

1. 掌握莪术中主要挥发性活性成分的化学结构和莪术油的定性定量分析方法。

2. 熟悉高效液相色谱法在挥发性成分分析中的应用。

【实验原理】

在挥发性成分分析中，气相色谱法是一种最常见的手段。但莪术油中的倍半萜类成分有的具有1，5－二烯结构（如牻牛儿酮、莪术二酮、呋喃二烯等），用气相色谱法测定易导致相关成分发生Cope重排，方法的准确性和重现性均受到影响。因此，在2015版《中国药典》一部中采用高效液相色谱法测定其含量来进行莪术油的质量控制。

【实验器材】

1. 仪器　高效液相色谱仪、C_{18}柱、容量瓶、移液管、展开缸等。

2. 试药与试剂　硅胶G薄层板、石油醚（60～90℃）、乙酸乙酯、冰醋酸、5%香草醛硫酸溶液、乙腈、无水乙醇、莪术油、牻牛儿酮对照品、呋喃二烯对照品、莪术醇对照品、莪术二酮对照品。

【实验步骤】

1. 定性分析　取本品4mg置1ml量瓶中，加石油醚（60～90℃）溶解至刻度，摇匀，即作为供试品溶液。另取莪术醇、牻牛儿酮和莪术二酮对照品，分别加石油醚（60～90℃）制成每1ml含0.5mg的溶液，作为对照品溶液。照薄层色谱法试验，吸取上述4种溶液各2μl，分别点于同一硅胶G薄层板上，以石油醚（60～90℃）－乙酸乙酯－冰醋酸（60∶5∶0.5）为展开剂，展开。取出，晾干，喷以5%香草醛硫酸溶液，在105℃加热至斑点显色清晰。供试品色谱中，在与对照品色谱相应的位置上，应显相同颜色的斑点。

2. 定量分析

（1）色谱条件　色谱柱：C_{18}柱；流动相：乙腈（A）－水（B），梯度洗脱（0～20分钟，60%A→95%A；21～35分钟，95%A）；检测波长：216nm；流速：1.0ml/min。

（2）对照品溶液的制备　取牻牛儿酮对照品及呋喃二烯对照品适量，精密称定，加无水乙醇制成每1ml含牻牛儿酮30μg、呋喃二烯50μg的混合溶液，即得。

（3）供试品溶液的制备　取本品0.1g，精密称定，置50ml量瓶中，加无水乙醇至刻度，摇匀，精密量取5ml，置25ml量瓶中，加无水乙醇至刻度，摇匀，滤过，取续滤液，即得。

（4）测定法　分别精密吸取对照品溶液和供试品溶液各5μl，注入液相色谱仪，测定，即得。

【实验记录】

1. 绘制定性薄层色谱图，记录莪术醇、牻牛儿酮和莪术二酮在本实验薄层色谱条件下的R_f值。

2. 用外标一点法计算莪术油中牻牛儿酮和呋喃二烯的含量。

【思考题】

1. 薄层色谱定性分析中，在展开剂中加入冰醋酸的目的是什么？

2. HPLC 定量分析莪术油中的活性成分，采用乙腈和水为流动相进行梯度洗脱的优点有哪些？

【相关资料】

1. 药材来源和化学成分 莪术为姜科植物蓬莪术 *Curcuma phaeocaulis* Val. 、广西莪术 *Curcuma kuangsiensis* S. G. Lee et C. F. 或温郁金 *Curcuma wenyujin* Y. H. Chen et C. Ling 的干燥根茎。后者习称“温莪术”。

莪术油为莪术（温莪术）经水蒸气蒸馏提取的挥发油。其主要成分为多种倍半萜类，包括呋喃二烯、莪术二酮、牻牛儿酮、榄香烯等。

《中国药典》（2015 年版）规定本品含牻牛儿酮（$C_{15}H_{22}O$）不得少于 7. 5%，含呋喃二烯（$C_{15}H_{20}O$）不得少于 10. 0%。

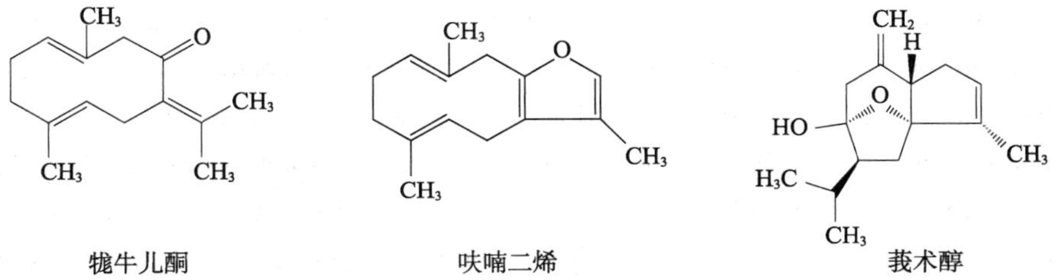

牻牛儿酮　　呋喃二烯　　莪术醇

2. 莪术油的理化性质 莪术油为浅棕色或深棕色的澄清液体；气特异，味苦而辛。在甲醇、乙醇、丙酮、乙酸乙酯、三氯甲烷、乙醚、甲苯或石油醚中易溶，在水中微溶。相对密度为 0. 970 ~ 0. 990；比旋度为 +20° ~ +25°；折光率为 1. 500 ~ 1. 510。

3. 功能与主治 莪术：具有破血行气，消积止痛的功效；用于癥瘕痞块，瘀血经闭，胸痹心痛，食积胀痛。

Experiment 3　The Qualitative and Quantitative Analysis of Zedoary Furmeric Oil

Purpose

1. Comprehend the chemical structures of the volatile active components in Zedoray Rhizome and the method of qualitative and quantitative analysis of Zedoary Furmeric oil.

2. Understand the use of HPLC in the determination of the volatile active components in TCM.

Principle

GC is a commonly used method in analysis of volatile oils. However, the sesquiterpenoids such as germacrone, curdione and furanodiene in Zedoary Furmeric Oil always have the structure of 1, 5 – diene. Previous work revealed that Cope rearrangement would easily occur during GC analysis for these compounds, which may affect the accuracy and reproducibility of the assay. Therefore, HPLC method is employed for the item of Assay to control the quality of Zedoary Furmeric Oil in Chinese Pharmacopeia (2015 edition).

Conditions

1. Apparatus HPLC instrument, C_{18} column, volumetric flask, pipette and developing chamber.

2. Reagents and materials Silica gel G thin layer plate, petroleum ether (60 ~ 90℃), ethyl acetate, glacial acetic acid, 5% vanillin sulfuric acid solution, acetonitrile, dehydrated ethanol, water, Zedoary Furmeric Oil, germacrone CRS, furanodiene CRS, curcumol CRS and Curdione CRS.

Experimental Procedure

1. Qualitative analysis Take 4mg of Zedoary Furmeric Oil in a 1ml volumetric flask, add petroleum ether (60 ~ 90℃) to volume and mix well. Dissolve a quantity of curcumol CRS, germacrone CRS and curdione CRS in petroleum ether (60 ~ 90℃), respectively, to produce a solution containing 0.5mg of each per ml as the reference solution. Carry out the method for thin layer chromatography, using silica gel G as the coating substance and a mixture of petroleum ether (60 ~ 90℃), ethyl acetate and glacial acetic acid (60:5:0.5) as the mobile phase. Apply separately 2μl of each of the above four solutions to the plate. After developing and removal of the plate, dry in air, spray with 5% vanillin in sulfuric acid and heat at 105℃ to the spots clear. The spots in the chromatogram obtained with the test solution correspond in position and color to the spots in chromatogram obtained with the reference solutions.

2. Quantitative analysis

(1) Chromatographic system Use octadecylsilane bonded silica gel as the stationary phase, acetonitrile as the mobile phase A and water as the mobile phase B, elute in gradient (0 ~ 20min, 60% A→95% A; 21 ~ 35min, 95% A); Wave length of detector: 216nm; Flow rate: 1.0ml/min.

(2) Reference solution Dissolve a quantity of germacrone CRS and furanodiene CRS, accurately weighed, in dehydrated ethanol to produce a mixture containing 30μg of germacrone and 50μg of furanodiene per ml as the reference solution.

(3) Test solution Dissolve 0.1g of Zedoary Furmeric Oil, accurately weighed, in a 50ml volumetric flask, dilute with dehydrated ethanol to volume and mix well. Measure accurately 5ml to a 25ml volumetric flask, dilute with dehydrated ethanol to volume and mix well, filter, use the successive filtrate as the test solution.

(4) Procedure Inject accurately 5μl of each of the reference solution and the test solution into the column, determine and calculate the content.

Experimental Records

1. Describe the chromatogram of thin layer chromatography, calculate the R_f values of curcumol, germacrone and curdione under the condition of this experiment.

2. Calculate the content of germacrone and furanodiene in Zedoary Furmeric Oil by one point external standard method.

Questions

1. What is the purpose of adding acetic acid to the developing agent?

2. What are the advantages of gradient elution by using acetonitrile and water as the mobile phase in HPLC assay?

Background Information

1. Origins and chemical constituents Curcumae Rhizoma is the dried rhizome of *Curcuma phaeocaulis* Valeton, *Curcuma kuangsiensis* S. G. Lee et C. F. Liang or *Curcuma wenyujin* Y. H. Chen et C. Ling (Fam. Zingiberaceae). The drug derived from the last species is commonly known as "Wen Ezhu".

Zedoary Furmeric Oil (Curcuma Oils) is the volatile oil obtained by steam distillation from Curcumae Rhizoma (Wenezhu). Main volatile active components from this drug are sesquiterpenoids, such as furanodiene, curdione, germacrone, elemene and so on.

It contains not less than 7.5 percent of germacrone ($C_{15}H_{22}O$) and 10.0 percent of furanodiene ($C_{15}H_{20}O$), according to the Chinese Pharmacopoeia (2015 edition).

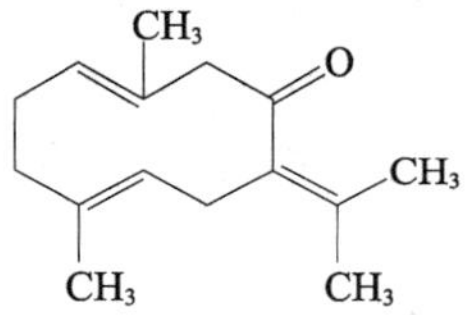
germacrone

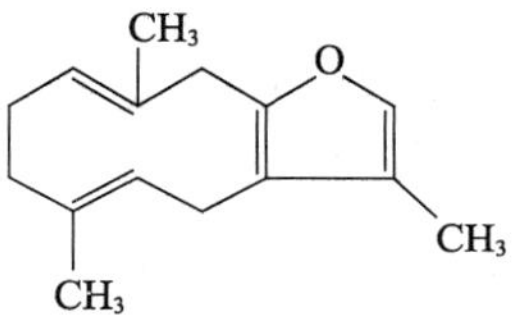
furanodien

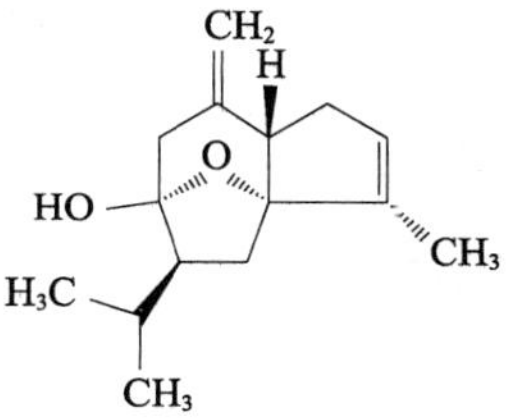
curcumol

2. Physical and chemical properties A pale brown or dark brown clear liquid; odour, characteristic; taste, slightly bitter and pungent.

Relative density: 0.97 ~ 0.990.

Specific optical rotation: +20° ~ +25°, in a solution of 50mg per ml in ethanol.

Reference index: 1.500 ~ 1.510.

Easily dissolve in methanol, ethanol, acetone, ethyl acetate, chloroform, ether, petroleum ether, benzene etc.. Slightly dissolve in water.

3. Actions and indications Curcumae Rhizoma: To move *qi* and break blood, eliminate accumulation and relieve pain. Used for aggregation – accumulation masses, glomus, blood – stasis amenorrhea, chest impediment and heart pain, food accumulation with distention pain.

实验四　麝香祛痛气雾剂中活性成分的定性定量分析

【实验目的】

1. 掌握中成药中樟脑、冰片、薄荷脑等成分的定性定量分析方法。

2. 熟悉气相色谱法在中药制剂分析中的应用。

【实验原理】

麝香祛痛气雾剂是由人工麝香、红花、樟脑、独活、冰片、龙血竭、薄荷脑、地黄、三七等九味药制成的具有活血祛瘀，舒经活络，消肿止痛之效的中药制剂。其中樟脑、薄荷脑、冰片为主要活性物质，均为挥发油类成分，故本实验采用气相色谱法鉴别和测定麝香祛痛气雾剂中这 3 种活性成分的含量。

【实验器材】

1. 仪器 气相色谱仪，氢火焰离子化检测器，DB－WAX 聚乙二醇（PEG）气相毛细管柱，微量进样器等。

2. 试剂与试药 无水乙醇，麝香祛痛气雾剂（市售），萘，樟脑对照品，薄荷脑对照品、冰片对照品。

【实验步骤】

1. 定性分析 取本品，照定量分析项下的方法试验，样品色谱中应呈现与樟脑对照品、薄荷脑对照品、冰片对照品色谱峰保留时间相同的色谱峰。

2. 定量分析 色谱条件与系统适应性实验：聚乙二醇 20000（PEG－20M）毛细管柱（柱长为 30m，内径为 0.53mm，膜厚度为 1.0μm），柱温为 160℃，检测器温度 230℃，检测器 FID，理论板数按樟脑峰计算应不低于 20000。

（1）校正因子测定 取萘适量，精密称定，加无水乙醇制成每 1ml 含 4mg 的溶液，作为内标溶液。另取樟脑对照品、薄荷脑对照品、冰片对照品各 30mg、10mg 、20mg，精密称定，置同一 50ml 量瓶中，精密加入内标溶液 5ml，加无水乙醇至刻度，摇匀，吸取 1μl，注入气相色谱仪，计算校正因子。

（2）样品溶液的配制 取本品，除去帽盖，冷却至 5℃，在铝盖上钻一小孔，插入连有干燥橡皮管的注射针头（勿与药液面接触），橡皮管另一端放入水中，待抛射剂缓缓排出后，除去铝盖，精密量取药液 1ml，置 50ml 量瓶中，精密加入内标溶液 5ml，加无水乙醇至刻度，摇匀，作为样品溶液。

（3）样品测定 吸取样品液 1μl，注入气相色谱仪，测定，即得。冰片以龙脑峰、异龙脑峰面积之和计算。

【实验记录】

根据下列公式分别计算樟脑、薄荷脑、冰片的含量：

$$(C_x) = f \cdot \frac{A_x}{A_s/C_s}$$

式中 A_s、A_x 为内标物质和样品液中樟脑、薄荷脑、冰片的峰面积；

C_s、C_x 为内标物质和样品液的浓度。

【思考题】

1. 用气相色谱法测定中药复方制剂中挥发性成分的优点？
2. 采用内标法计算含量的优点是什么？

【相关资料】

1. 处方组成 麝香祛痛气雾剂为非定量阀门气雾剂，在耐压容器中的药液为橙红色澄清液体；气芳香。由人工麝香 0.33g，红花 1g，樟脑 30g，独活 1g，冰片 20g，龙血竭 0.33g，薄荷脑 10g，地黄 20g，三七 0.33g 制成。

2. 有效成分及其理化性质 本品有效成分为樟脑、薄荷脑、冰片，2015 版《中国药典》规定，本品（气相色谱法）每 1ml 中含樟脑应为 25.5～34.5mg，薄荷脑应为 8.5～11.5mg，含冰片应为 17.0～ 23.0mg。

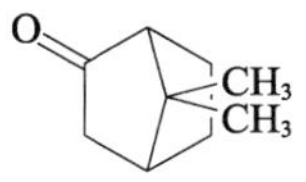

樟脑

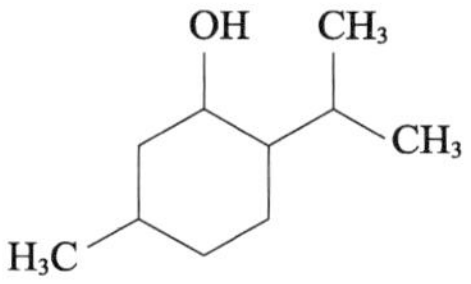

薄荷脑

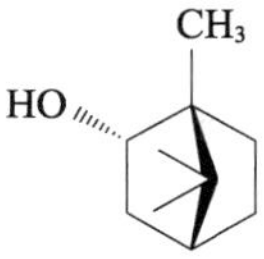

冰片

樟脑（2－莰酮）的分子量为 152.23。无色至白色半透明块状或粉末，有樟木气味，熔点 174～179℃。沸点 204℃，－1.5～＋1.5°，微溶于水，溶于乙醇、醚、三氯甲烷、二硫化碳等多种有机溶剂。

薄荷脑的分子量为 156.27。无色针状或棱柱状结晶或白色结晶性粉末，有薄荷的特殊香气，熔点 42～44℃。比旋度－49°～－50°，微溶于水，极易溶于乙醇、三氯甲烷、乙醚。

冰片（合成龙脑）的分子量为 154.25。无色透明或白色半透明的片状松脆结晶，气清香，熔点 205～210℃，几乎不溶于水，易溶于乙醇、三氯甲烷或乙醚。

3. 功能与主治　活血祛瘀，舒经活络，消肿止痛。用于各种跌打损伤，瘀血肿痛，风湿瘀阻，关节疼痛。

（刘丽芳）

Experiment 4　The Qualitative and Quantitative Analysis of Active Components in Shexiang Qutong Aerosol

Purpose

1. Comprehend the qualitative and quantitative analysis method of camphor, menthol, (±)－borneol and (±)－isoborneol in the Chinese patent medicine.

2. Understand the application of gas chromatography in the analysis of Chinese medicine preparation.

Principle

Shexiang Qutong Aerosol is a traditional Chinese medicine preparation composed of Moschus Artifactus, Carthami Flos, Camphora, Angelicae Pubescentis Radix, Borneolum synthe－ticum, Dracaenae Combodianae Resina, *l*－menthol, Rehmanniac Radix, and Notoginseng Radix Rhizoma. The preparation can active blood, resolve stasis, sooth meridians, harmonize collaterals, alleviate edema and relieve pain. Camphor, *l*－menthol and borneol are the main active components contained in this preparation, and can be gasified in a certain temperature. Therefore, GC method is used to determine the content of these active constituents in this preparation.

Conditions

1. Apparatus　Gas chromatograph, flame ionization detector, DB－WAX PEG capillary column, mycrosyringe.

2. Reagents and materials Shexiang Qutong Aerosol (commercially available), naphthalene, camphor CRS, menthol CRS, (±) -borneol and (±) -isoborneol CRS, dehydrated ethanol.

Experimental Procedure

1. Qualitative analysis Carry out the same method under Quantitative analysis, the retention times of the peaks in the chromatogram obtained with the test solution correspond to the peaks in the chromatogram obtained with camphor CRS, menthol CRS, (±) -borneol and (±) -isoborneol CRS.

2. Quantitative analysis

(1) Chromatographic system and system suitability Use a macrogol-20000 (PEG-20M) fused quartz capillary column (0.53mm in internal diameter, 30 meter long and 1.0μm film thickness) as the stationary phase, maintain the column temperature at 160℃. Use flame ionization detector (FID). The number of theoretical plates of the column is not less than 20000, calculated with reference to the peak of camphor.

(2) Calculation of correction factor Dissolve a quantity of naphthalene, accurately weighed, in dehydrated ethanol to prepare a solution containing 4mg per ml, as the internal standard solution, Dissolve 30mg of camphor CRS, 10mg of menthol CRS and 20mg of (±)-borneol and (±) -isoborneol CRS, accurately weighed, in a same 50ml volumetric flask, add accurately 1ml of the internal standard solution, dilute with dehydrated ethanol to volume, and mix well. Inject 1μl of the solution into column, calculate the correction factor.

(3) Test solution Remove the cover of the container, cool to 5℃. On the aluminum cover of the container punch a hole and insert an injection needle with a dry rubber into the container (do not contact the surface of the liquid). The other end of the rubber tubing is inserted into water, allow the propellant to expel gently completely, remove the aluminum cover. Measure accurately 1ml of the drug liquid, to a 50ml volumetric flask, add accurately 5ml of the internal standard solution, dilute with dehydrated ethanol to volume, mix well, as the test solution.

(4) Procedure Inject 1μl of the test solution into the column, determine and calculate the contents.

Experimental Records

From the values obtained, calculate the content of camphor, menthol and borneol as follows:

$$(C_x) = f \cdot \frac{A_x}{A_s/C_s}$$

In which,

A_x = peak area of sample;

A_s = peak area of the internal standard;

C_x = concentration of sample;

C_s = concentration of the internal standard.

Questions

1. What are the advantages of analysis of volatile constituents in compound Chinese medicinal preparation by gas chromatography?

2. What is the advantage of using internal standard method to calculate the content?

Background Information

1. Ingredients This drug is an aerosol with non - metered - dose valve system, the drug liquid in the pressure - resistant container is a clear, orangish - red liquid with aromatic odour. The ingredients are Moschus Artifactus 0. 33g, Carthami Flos 1g, Camphora 30g, Angelicae Pubescentis Radix 1g, Borneolum synthe - ticum 20g, Dracaenae Combodianae Resina 0. 33g, *l* - menthol 10g, Rehmanniae Radix 20g and Notoginseng Radix Rhizoma 0. 33g.

2. The physical and chemical properties of three active components The main active components are camphor, menthol, (±) - borneol and (±) - isoborneol in this sample. According to the Chinese pharmacopoeia (2015 edition), the contents of three components in the sample should be: camphor: 25. 5 ~ 34. 5mg/ml; menthol: 8. 5 ~ 11. 5mg/ml; (±) - borneol and (±) - isoborneol: 17. 0 ~ 23. 0mg/ml.

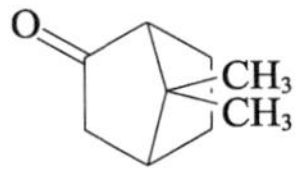

camphor

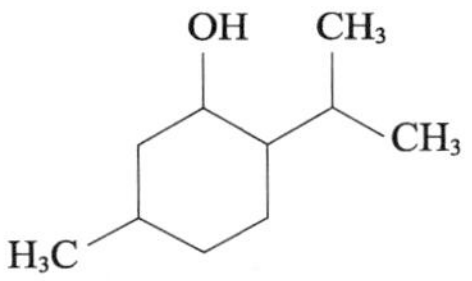

menthol

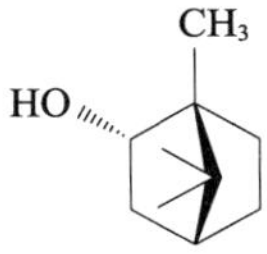

borneol

The molecular weight of camphor is 152. 23, colorless to white translucent block or powder, camphor odor. Melting point: 174 ~ 179℃, boiling point: 204℃, specific rotation: −1. 5 ~ +1. 5°, slightly soluble in water, soluble in organic solvents, such as ethanol, ether, chloroform, carbon disulfide and so on.

The molecular weight of menthol is 156. 27, colorless needle or prismatic crystals or white crystalline powder, special mint aroma. Melting point: 42 ~ 44℃, specific rotation: −49 ~ −50°, slightly soluble in water, easily soluble in alcohol, chloroform and ether.

The molecular weight of borneol is 154. 25. Colorless transparent or translucent white flaky crunchy crystals, fragrance. Melting point: 205 ~ 210℃, almost insoluble in water, freely soluble in ethanol, chloroform or ether.

3. Actions and indications To active blood, resolve stasis, sooth meridians, harmonize collaterals, alleviate edema and relieve pain. Used for all kinds of injuries from falls and fights, caused by swelling pain due to static bloodswelling caused by static blood, wind - dampness stasis and obstruction, and joints pain.

(Lifang Liu)

第六章
其他类成分的分析

实验一　高效液相色谱法测定女贞子中特女贞苷的含量

【实验目的】

1. 掌握环烯醚萜类成分的结构特性。

2. 掌握高效液相色谱法测定环烯醚萜类成分的原理。

【实验原理】

特女贞苷为女贞子的主要有效成分，属于环烯醚萜类成分，由于其结构中存在共轭双键，因此具有紫外吸收。本实验以特女贞苷作为对照品，采用高效液相色谱法测定药材中特女贞苷的含量。

【实验器材】

1. 仪器　高效液相色谱仪，微量进样器，超声清洗仪等。

2. 试剂与试药　特女贞苷对照品，女贞子药材粉末，甲醇，乙醇，水。

【实验步骤】

1. 色谱条件与系统适用性试验　以十八烷基硅烷键合硅胶为填充剂；以甲醇－水（40∶60）为流动相；检测波长为224nm。理论板数按特女贞苷峰计算应不低于4000。

2. 对照品溶液的制备　取特女贞苷对照品适量，精密称定，加甲醇制成每1ml含0.25mg的溶液，即得。

3. 供试品溶液的制备　取本品粉末（过三号筛）约0.5g，精密称定，置具塞锥形瓶中，精密加入稀乙醇50ml，称定重量，加热回流1小时，放冷，再称定重量，用稀乙醇补足减失的重量，摇匀，滤过，取续滤液，即得。

4. 测定法　分别精密吸取对照品溶液5μl与供试品溶液10μl，注入液相色谱仪，测定，即得。

【实验记录】

1. 记录实验结果，实验现象及出现问题并讨论。

2. 计算女贞子中特女贞苷的含量，并比对其他5个实验小组的结果，计算相对平均偏差。

【思考题】

环烯醚萜类成分的结构特点是什么？

【相关资料】

1. 药材来源　本品为木犀科植物女贞 *Ligustrum lucidum* Ait. 的干燥成熟果实。冬季果实成熟时采收，除去枝叶，稍蒸或置沸水中略烫后，干燥；或直接干燥。

2. 女贞子的化学成分　特女贞苷的分子量为686.656，类白色结晶粉末，熔点152～155℃，密度1.53。易溶于甲醇，乙醇，不溶于石油醚。主要含有女贞子苷、特女贞苷、女贞子素、橄榄苦苷、女贞子酸、齐墩果酸、白华醇及女贞子多糖等。

《中国药典》（2015年版）规定特女贞苷的含量不得少于0.70%（高效液相法）。

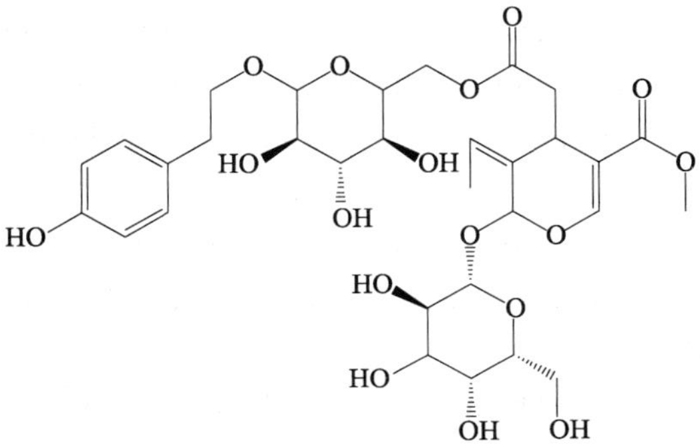

特女贞苷

3. 功能与主治　滋补肝肾，明目乌发。用于肝肾阴虚，眩晕耳鸣，腰膝酸软，须发早白，目暗不明，内热消渴，骨蒸潮热。

Experiment 1　The Determination of Specnuezhenide in Ligustri Lucidi Fructus by HPLC

Purpose

1. Comprehend the properties of iridoids and its quantitative methods.

2. Comprehend the application of HPLC in the determination of iridoid compounds.

Principles

Specnuezhenide is the major bioactive compound of Ligustri Lucidi Fructus. In this experiment, we will determine the content of specnuezhenide in this Chinese herb. We can identify the peak of specnuezhenide in the sample through comparing the retention time with reference. Then, the content of specnuezhenide in the sample can be calculated by the external standard method.

Conditions

1. Apparatus　HPLC instrument, C_{18} column, ultrasonicate cleaner, etc..

2. Reagents and materials　Ligustri Lucidi Fructus, specnuezhenide CRS, methanol,

ethanol and water.

Experimental Procedure

1. Chromatographic system and system suitability Use octadecylsilane bonded silica gel as the stationary phase and a mixture of methanol and water (40∶60) as the mobile phase. The wavelength of the detector is 224nm. The number of theoretical plates of the column is not less than 4000, calculated with reference to the peak of specnuezhenide.

2. Reference solution Weigh accurately 6.25mg of specnuezhenide CRS in a 25ml volumetric flask, dissolve and dilute with methanol to volume, mix well to produce a solution containing 0.25mg of specnuezhenide per ml as the reference solution.

3. Test solution Weigh accurately 0.5g of the powder (through No. 3 sieve) in a conical flask with plug, add about 50ml of dilute ethanol and weigh, heat under reflux for 1 hour, cool, weigh it again and replenish the loss of solvent with dilute ethanol, shake well and filter, use the filtrate as the reference solution.

4. Procedure Accurately inject 5μl of the reference solution and 10μl of the test solution, respectively, into the column, determine and calculate the content.

Experiment records

1. Record the process and problems occurred during the experiment, and discuss them briefly.

2. Calculate the content of specnuezhenide in Ligustri Lucidi Fructus and calculate the relative standard deviation (RSD) by comparing with the results of other 5 groups.

Questions

What is the structure characteristic of iridoid?

Background Information

1. Origins Ligustri Lucidi Fructus is the dried ripe fruit of *Ligustrum lucidum* Ait. (Oleaceae). The ripe fruit is collected in winter, by removing from leafy branches, steamed or treated with boiling water for a few minutes, then dried; or dried directly without treatment to obtain Ligustri Lucidi Fructus.

The major ingredients of Ligusri Lucidi Fructus are including nuezhenide, specnuezhenide, ligustrin, oleuropein, nuezhenidic acid, oleanolic, botulin and polysaccharide.

2. Chemical constituents Specnuezhenide ($C_{31}H_{42}O_{17}$): The molecular weight is 686.656; cherry red needle crystal (methanol); the melting point is 152 ~ 155℃; It is insoluble in petroleum ether while it is soluble in alcohol or ethanol.

3. Actions and indications To nourish the liver and kidney, improve vision and blacken hairs. Used for liver – kidney yin deficiency, dizziness and tinnitus, soreness and weakness in the low back and knees, premature graying, dim and blurred vision, interior heat wasting – thirst, bone – steaming and tidal fever.

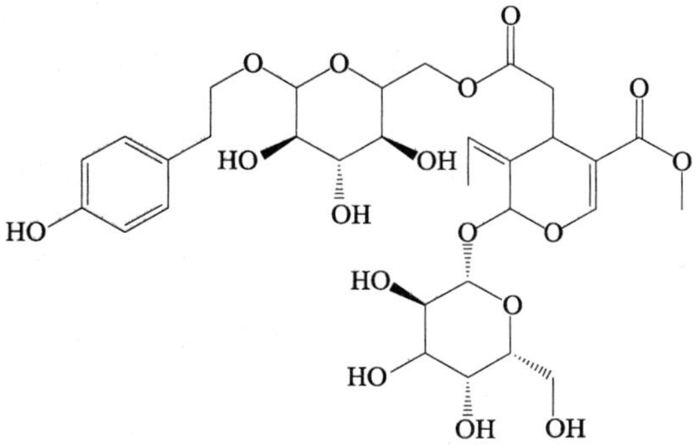

specnuezhenide

实验二　HPLC 法测定厚朴中木脂素类成分含量

【实验目的】

1. 掌握厚朴酚及和厚朴酚的结构特征和含量测定的方法。
2. 掌握高效液相色谱法在木脂素类多成分含量测定中的应用。

【实验原理】

厚朴酚与和厚朴酚是厚朴中的主要活性成分，按结构类型分类属于木脂素类成分。由于具有较高的共轭结构，二者在 294nm 处有较强的紫外吸收。因此，本实验以厚朴酚及和厚朴酚作为对照品，采用高效液相色谱法测定了药材中厚朴酚、和厚朴酚的含量。

【实验器材】

1. 仪器　高效液相色谱仪，微量进样器，超声波清洗器等。

2. 试剂与试药　厚朴酚与和厚朴酚对照品，厚朴药材粉末，甲醇，水。

【实验步骤】

1. 色谱条件与系统适应性试验　以十八烷基硅烷键合硅胶为填充剂；以甲醇－水（78∶22）为流动相；检测波长为 294nm。理论板数按厚朴酚峰计算应不低于 3800。

2. 对照品溶液的制备　取厚朴酚对照品、和厚朴酚对照品各 1.0mg，精密称定，置于 2.0ml 量瓶，加甲醇至刻度。

3. 供试品溶液的制备　取本品粉末（过三号筛）约 0.2g，精密称定，置具塞锥形瓶中，精密加入甲醇 25ml，摇匀，超声提取 25 分钟滤过，滤液置 100ml 量瓶中，重复提取 2 次，合并滤液，加甲醇至刻度，摇匀，即得。

4. 测定法　分别精密吸取对照品溶液与供试品溶液各 1μl，注入液相色谱仪，测定，计算。

【实验记录】

1. 记录实验结果，计算厚朴中厚朴酚与和厚朴酚的含量。
2. 结合邻近 4 个实验小组的结果，计算相对平均偏差（n＝5）。

【思考题】

木脂素类成分的结构特点是什么？

【相关资料】

1. 药材来源 本品为木兰科植物厚朴 *Magnolia officinalis Rehd.* et Wils. 或凹叶厚朴 *Magnolia officinalis Rehd.* et Wils. 的干燥干皮、根皮及枝皮。4 ~6 月剥取，根皮和枝皮直接阴干；干皮置沸水中微煮后，堆置阴湿处，“发汗”至内表面变紫褐色或棕褐色时，蒸软，取出，卷成筒状，干燥。

2. 厚朴的化学成分 厚朴主要含有厚朴酚（magnolol）及和厚朴酚（hohokiol），尚有厚朴三酚 B（magnatriol），厚朴醛 B、D（magnaldehyde B，D）及木质素 F（magnolignan F）。

《中国药典》规定厚朴中含厚朴酚与和厚朴酚的总量不得少于 2.0%。（用高效液相色法）

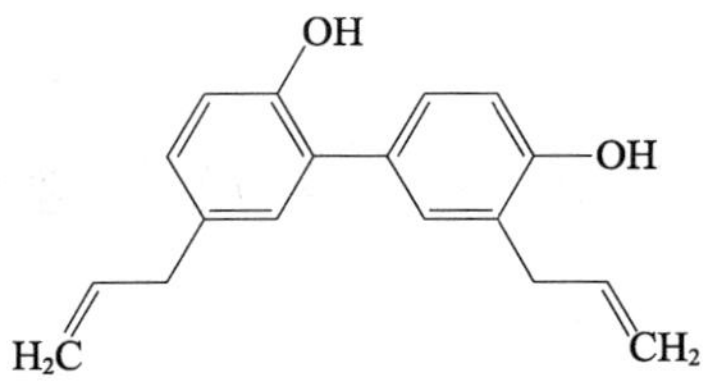

厚朴酚

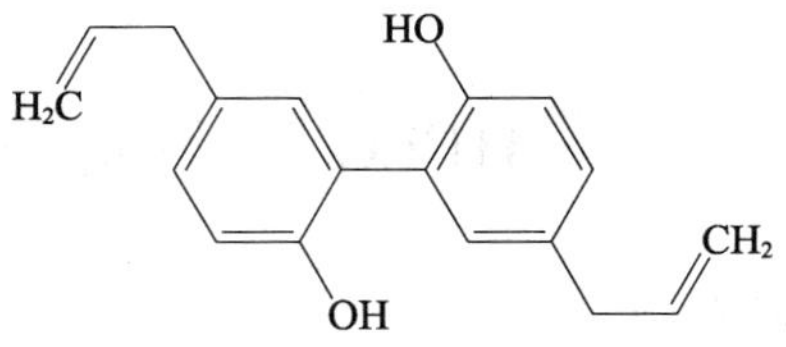

和厚朴酚

3. 功能与主治 燥湿消痰，下气除满。用于湿滞伤中，脘痞吐泻，食积气滞，腹胀便秘，痰饮喘咳。

Experiment 2 The Determination of Lignins in Magnoliae Officinalis Cortex by HPLC

Purpose

1. Comprehend the properties of magnolol and honokiol.

2. Comprehend the application of HPLC in determination of lignins.

Principles

Both magnolmol and honokiol are the main bioactive compounds of Magnoliae Officinalis Cortex. In this experiment, we will determine the content of magnolol and honokiol in Magnoliae Officinalis Cortex. We can identify the peak of magnolol and honokiol in the sample through comparing the retention time with reference. Then, the content of magnolol and honokiol in the sample can be calculated by the external standard method.

Conditions

1. Apparatus HPLC instrument, C_{18} column, ultrasonicate cleaner, etc..

2. Reagents and materials Magnoliae Officinalis Cortex, magnolol CRS, honokiol CRS, methanol and water.

Experimental Procedure

1. Chromatographic system and system suitability Use octadecylsilane bonded silica gel as the stationary phase and a mixture of methanol and water (65∶35) as the mobile phase, the flow rate is 1. 0ml/min, the wavelength of the detector is 294nm. The number of theoretical plates of the column is not less than 3800, calculated with reference to the peak of magnolol.

2. Reference solution Weigh accurately 1. 0mg of magnolol CRS and honokiol CRS, respectively, in 2. 0ml of methanol to produce two solutions containing 0. 5mg of each per ml.

3. Test solution Weigh accurately 0. 2g of the sample powder (through No. 3 sieve) to a 50ml conical flask, add 25ml of methanol, ultrasonicate for 15 minutes and filter. Transfer the fiitrate to a 100ml volumetric flask. Extract the residue in the same manner for 2 times. Combine the extracts to the same volumetric flask, dilute with methanol to volume and mix well.

4. Procedure Accurately inject 10μl of each of the reference solution and the test solution respectively into the column, determine and calculate the content.

Experiment records

1. Record the results of this experiment, and calculate the content of magnolol and honokiol in Magnoliae Officinalis Cortex.

2. Calculate the relative standard deviation (RSD) of the contents by comparing with your 4 neighboring groups' data ($n = 5$).

Questions

What is the structure characteristic of lignins?

Background Information

1. Origins Magnoliae Officinalis Cortex is the dried stem bark of *Magnolia officinalis* Rehd. et Wils. or *Magnolia officinalis* Rehd. et Wils. var. *biloba* Rehd. et Wils. (Magnoliaceae). The stem bark is collected in the spring and summer, and then boiled in water until soft, then piled in a wet place until its inner surface and the surface of the transverse section purplish - brown or brown in colour and shiny or showing luster, then further softened by steaming, rolled and dried to obtain Magnoliae Officinalis Cortex.

2. Chemical constituents The main ingredients of Magnoliae Officinalis Cortex are including magnolol, hohokiol, magnatriol, magnaldehyde B, D and magnolignan F.

The sample contains not less than 2. 0% of the total content of magnolol ($C_{18}H_{18}O_2$) and honokiol ($C_{18}H_{18}O_2$), calculated with reference to the dried drug (Ch. P. , 2015 edition, by HPLC).

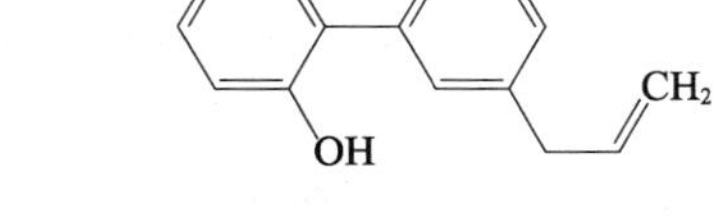

magnolol

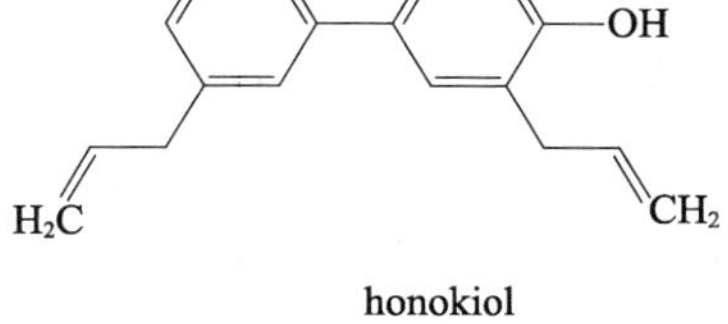

honokiol

3. Actions and indications To dry dampness and resolve phlegm, direct *qi* downward to disperse fullness. Used for dampness stagnation, vomiting and diarrhea, food accumulation and *qi* stagnation, abdominal distension and constipation, panting and cough caused by phlegm – fluid retention.

实验三 高效液相指纹图谱法鉴定何首乌药材

【实验目的】

1. 了解液相指纹图谱在中药材鉴定中的应用。
2. 掌握相对保留时间的计算。

【实验原理】

中药化学指纹图谱（chemical fingerprint），它是利用中药中次生代谢产物（化学物质，或称化学成分）的多样性，应用色谱与光谱技术可以得到一组反映其次生代谢产物的图像，通过比较不同样品间这些图像的共性与差异，用于中药的品种鉴定与品质评价。其中应用最广泛的是高效液相色谱（HPLC）指纹图谱。

【实验器材】

1. 仪器 高效液相色谱仪，超声波清洗器，C_{18}柱（4.6×250mm）等。

2. 试药与试剂 何首乌药材粉末，2，3，5，4'–四羟基二苯乙烯苷–2–*O*–*β*–*D*葡萄糖苷对照品，乙腈，甲醇，水。

【实验步骤】

1. 色谱条件与系统适应性实验 色谱柱：C_{18}柱（4.6×250mm）；流动相：乙腈为流动相A，0.1磷酸溶液为流动相B，按以下程序进行梯度洗脱：

时间（分钟）	流动相A（%，v/v）	流动相B（%，v/v）
0~35	90→60	10→40
35~55	60→0	40→100
55~70	0	100

检测波长：320nm，流速：1ml/min。

吸取对照品溶液10μl，注入液相色谱仪，重复5次。系统适用性的参数要求如下：2，3，5，4'–四羟基二苯乙烯苷–2–*O*–*β*–*D*葡萄糖苷的峰面积相对标准偏差应不得大于3.0%，保留时间的相对标准偏差应不大于2.0%；理论塔板数不得低于10000。

2. 对照品溶液的制备 精密称取2，3，5，4'–四羟基二苯乙烯苷–2–*O*–*β*–*D*葡萄糖苷对照品5mg，加甲醇制成每1ml含50μg的标准溶液。

3. 供试品溶液的制备 取10批样品，每个批次取粉末（过三号筛）0.2g，精密称定，置具塞锥形瓶中，加入丙酮25ml，密塞，称定重量，超声处理60分钟。放冷，再称定重量，用丙酮补足减失的重量，摇匀，滤过。精密量取续滤液10ml，置250ml圆底烧瓶中，旋转蒸发至干，用2ml甲醇溶解，过微孔滤膜，取续滤液，作为供试品溶液。

4. 测定法　吸取对照品和供试品溶液10μl注入液相色谱仪，记录图谱。测定指标成分2，3，5，4'－四羟基二苯乙烯苷－2－O－β－D葡萄糖苷的保留时间，通过比对10批样品找出共有峰，记录各共有峰的保留时间，并根据以下公式计算相对保留时间。

$$相对保留时间=\frac{特征峰保留时间}{参照峰保留时间}$$

【实验记录】

1. 扼要说明操作步骤及实验结果。
2. 找出共有峰，计算相对保留时间。

【思考题】

1. 在仪器操作过程中，应重点注意哪些方面。
2. 指纹图谱法在中药材鉴定中的应用中有哪些优势。

【相关资料】

1. 药材来源　本品为蓼科植物何首乌 *Polygonum multiflorum* Thunb. 的干燥块根。秋、冬二季叶枯萎时采挖，削去两端，洗净，个大的切成块，干燥。

2. 蓼科植物所含常见化学成分　没食子酸、儿茶素、虎杖苷、二苯乙烯苷、番泻苷B、番泻苷A、白藜芦醇、芦荟大黄素、大黄酸、大黄素、大黄酚、大黄素甲醚以及大黄素－8－O－β－D－葡萄糖苷等。

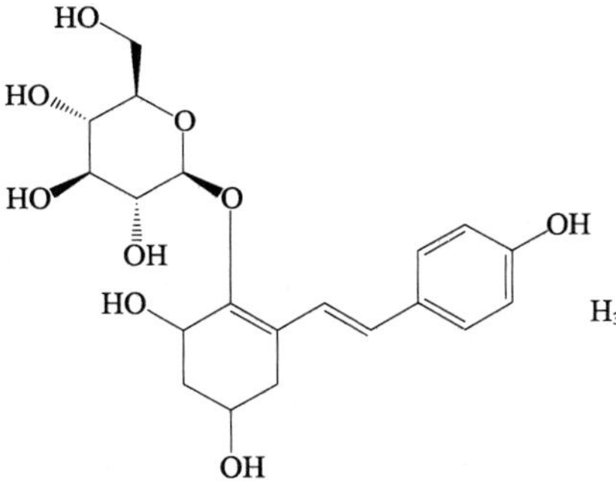

2,3,5,4'-四羟基二苯乙烯苷

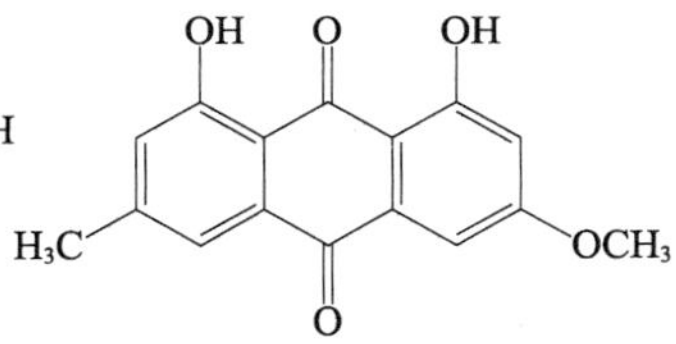

大黄素甲醚

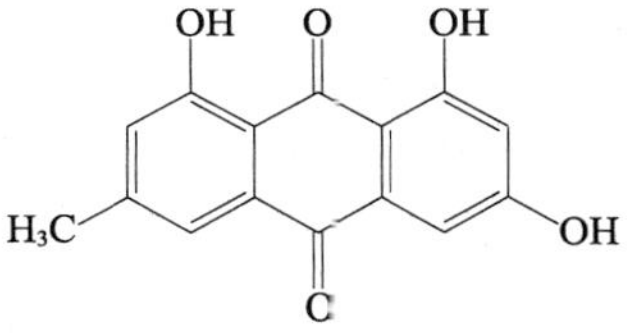

大黄素

3. 功能与主治　解毒，消痈，截疟，润肠通便。用于疮痈，瘰疬，风疹瘙痒，久疟体虚，肠燥便秘。

Experiment 3　The Identification of Polygoni Multiflori Radix by HPLC Fingerprinting

Purpose

1. Comprehend the calculation of relative retention time.
2. Know about the application of HPLC fingerprinting method in identification of traditional Chinese medicine.

Principles

The chemical fingerprint is based on the diversity of secondary metabolites in traditional

Chinese medicine, and using chromatographic and spectroscopic techniques to obtain a set of images reflecting its secondary metabolites. The similarities and differences of these images among different samples can be used for cultivar identification and quality evaluation of traditional Chinese medicine. HPLC fingerprint is the most extensive application of all the techniques.

Conditions

1. Apparatus HPLC instrument, C_{18} column, ultrasonicate cleaner, etc..

2. Reagents and materials 2, 3, 5, 4' – tetrahydroxystilbene – 2 – O – β – D – glucoside CRS, Polygoni Multiflori Radix, acetonitrile, methanol and water.

Experimental Procedure

1. Chromatographic system and system suitability Use octadecylsilane bonded silica gel as the stationary phase, acetonitrile as the mobile phase A, 0. 1% solution of phosphoric acid as the mobile phase B, elute in gradient as following:

Time (min)	Mobile phase A (per cent, v/v)	Mobile phase B (per cent, v/v)
0 – 35	90→60	10→40
35 – 55	60→0	40→100
55 – 70	0	100

As detectora spectrophotometer set at 320nm. The flow rate is 1. 0ml/min.

Perform at least five replicate injections each with 10μl of reference solution. The requirements of the system suitability parameters are as follows: the RSD value of the peak area of 2, 3, 5, 4' – tetrahydroxystilbene – 2 – O – β – D – glucoside should be not more than 3. 0%. The RSD value of the retention time of 2, 3, 5, 4' – tetrahydroxystilbene – 2 – O – β – D – glucoside peak should be not more than 2. 0%. The Rvalue between peak 1 and the closest peak in the chromatogram of the test solution should be not less than 1. 5. The number of theoretical plates of the column is not less than 50000, calculated with reference to the peak of 2, 3, 5, 4' tetrahydroxystilbene – 2 – O – β – D – glucoside.

2. Reference solution Weigh accurately a quantity of 2, 3, 5, 4' – tetrahydroxystilbene – 2 – O – β – D – glucoside CRS, dissolve in methanol to produce a solution containing 50μg per ml , mix well, as the reference solution.

3. Test solution Collected 10 batches of sample, weigh accurately 0. 2g of the powder (through No. 3 sieve) in a stopper conical flask, add accurately 25ml of acetone, stopper tightly and weigh, ultrasonicate for 20minutes, weigh again, replenish the loss solvent with acetone, filter. Transfer accurately 10ml of the successive filtrate to a 250ml round – bottomed flask. Evaporate the filtrate to dryness in vacuum. Dissolve the residue in 2ml of methanol, mix well and filter through a 0. 45mm millipore memberine, and use the successive filtrate as the test solution.

Procedure Separately inject 2, 3, 5, 4' – tetrahydroxystilbene – 2 – O – β – D – glucoside Std – FP and 10 batches of the test solution (10L each) into the HPLC system and record the chromatograms. Measure the retention times of 2, 3, 5, 4' – tetrahydroxystilbene – 2 – *O* – *β* – D – glucoside peak in the chromatograms of the corresponding Std – FP. By comparative analysis of chromatograms of the test solutions to find out common characteristic peaks of Radix Polygoni Multiflori and record the retention times. Under the same HPLC conditions, identify 2, 3, 5, 4' – tetrahydroxystilbene – 2 – *O* – *β* – D – glucoside peak in the chromatogram of the test solution by comparing their retention times with those in the chromatograms of the corresponding Std – FP. The retention times of 2, 3, 5, 4' – tetrahydroxystilbene – 2 – *O* – *β* – D – glucoside peaks in the chromatograms of the test solution and the corresponding Std – FP should not differ from their counterparts by more than 2.0% . Calculate the RRTs of the characteristic peaks by using the equation as

$$RRT = \frac{\text{Retention time of the characteristic peak}}{\text{Retention time of the marker peak}}$$

Experiment records

1. Describe briefly about the processes of this experiment.

2. Plot the standard curve and calculate the regression equation and relative factor.

Questions

1. What should be paid attention to in the operation of the instrument?

2. How to identify common characteristic peaks of Polygoni Multiflori Radix and calculate the RRTs?

Background Information

1. Origins Polygoni Multiflori Radix is the dried tuberous root of *Polygonum multiflorum* Thunb. (Polygonaceae). The tuberous root is collected in autumn and winter when the leaves wither. Both pointed ends are cut off, washed clean, and the large ones are cut into pieces and dried.

2. Chemical constituents Gallic acid, epicatechin, piceid, 2, 3, 5, 4' – tetrahydroxystilbene – 2 – *O* – *β* – D – glucoside, sennoside B, sennoside A, resveratrol, aloe – emodin, rhein, emodin, chrysophanol, physcion and emodin – 8 – *O* – *β* – D – glucoside.

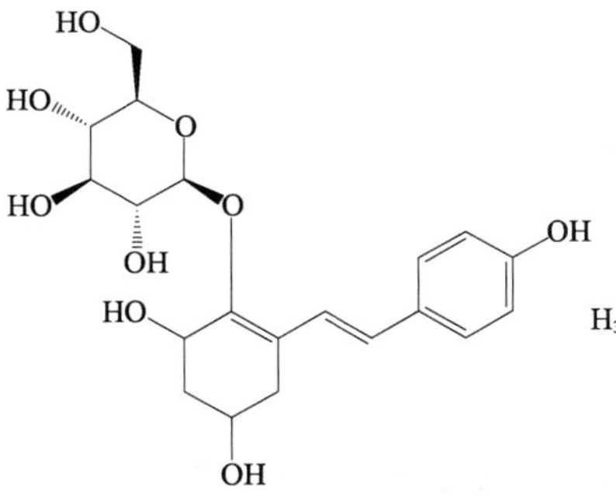

2,3,5,4'-tetrahydroxystilbene-2-O-*β*-D-glucoside

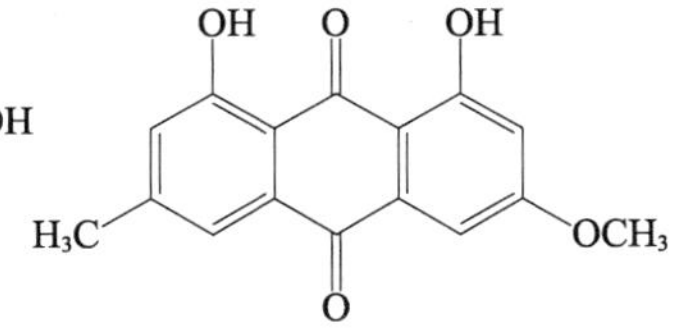

physcion

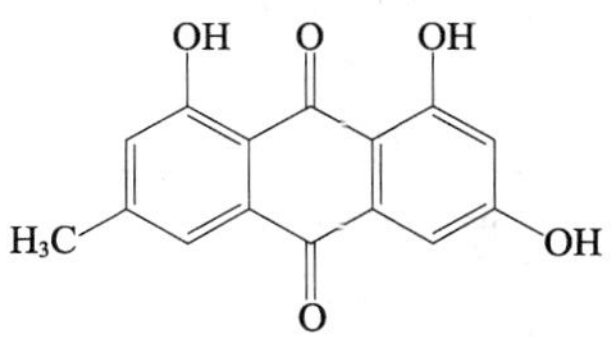

emodin

3. Actions and indications To remove toxin, disperse abscesses, interrupt malaria, and moisten the intestines to relax the bowels. Used for sore and abscess, scrofula, itching caused by rubella, weak constitution caused by long - term malaria, constipation caused by intestinal dryness.

实验四　高效液相色谱法测定金银花中绿原酸的含量

【实验目的】

1. 掌握绿原酸的结构特性及含量测定方法。

2. 掌握高效液相色谱法在有机酸含量测定中的应用。

【实验原理】

金银花是常用中药材，含有有机酸，环烯醚萜和黄酮等多种活性成分，其中，绿原酸是评价该药材质量的重要指标性成分之一，我国药典规定金银花中含绿原酸的量不得少于1.5%。本实验将采用高效液相色谱法测定金银花中绿原酸的含量。

【实验器材】

1. 仪器　高效液相色谱仪、紫外检测器、微量进样器、超声仪。

2. 试药与试剂　金银花药材粉末、绿原酸对照品、乙腈、纯水、磷酸。

【实验步骤】

1. 色谱条件与系统适用性试验　以十八烷基硅烷键合硅胶为填充剂；以乙腈-0.4%磷酸溶液（13:87）为流动相；检测波长为327nm。理论板数按绿原酸峰计算应不低于1000。

2. 对照品溶液的制备　取绿原酸对照品适量，精密称定，置棕色量瓶中，加50%甲醇制成每1ml含1mg的溶液，即得（10℃以下保存）。精密吸取母液适量，依次用50%甲醇配置为系列标准溶液20、40、60、200、400μg/ml。

3. 供试品溶液的制备　取本品粉末（过四号筛）约0.5g，精密称定，置具塞锥形瓶中，精密加入50%甲醇50ml，称定重量，超声处理（功率250W，频率35kHz）30分钟，放冷，再称定重量，用50%甲醇补足减失的重量，摇匀，滤过，精密量取续滤液5ml，置25ml棕色量瓶中，加50%甲醇至刻度，摇匀，即得。

4. 测定法　分别精密吸取上述对照品溶液与供试品溶液各10μl，注入液相色谱仪，测定，即得。

【实验记录】

1. 记录实验结果，绘制标准曲线图并计算回归方程和相关系数。

2. 计算金银花中绿原酸的含量。

【思考题】

测定有机酸类化学成分的方法有哪些？

【相关资料】

1. 药材来源　金银花为忍冬科植物忍冬 *Lonicera japonica* Thunb. 的干燥花蕾或带初开的花。夏初花开放前采收，干燥。具有清热解毒，疏散风热的功效。用于痈肿疔疮，喉痹，丹毒，热毒血痢，风热感冒，温病发热。

2. 金银花中的化学成分　绿原酸（$C_{16}H_{18}O_9$）：分子量为354.31。熔点207～

209℃。易溶于乙醇及丙酮，极微溶于醋酸乙酯，难溶于三氯甲烷、乙醚、苯等亲脂性有机溶剂。

绿原酸是由咖啡酸与奎尼酸生成的缩酚酸，是植物体在有氧呼吸过程中经莽草酸途径产生的一种苯丙素类化合物。具有抗氧化及降低饮食后糖进入血液循环的速率的作用。

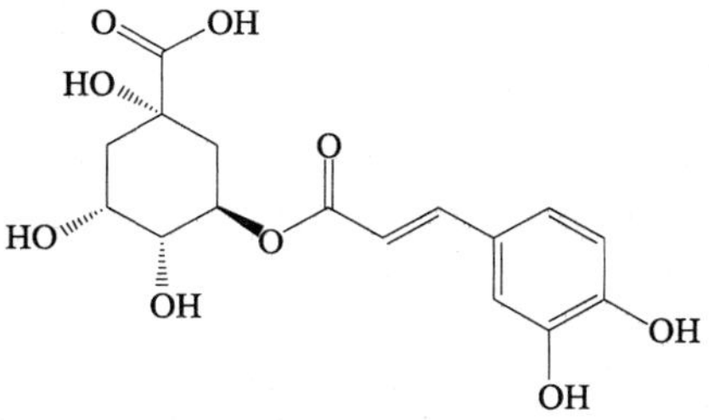

绿原酸

3. 功能与主治　清热解毒，疏散风热。用于痈肿疔疮，喉痹，丹毒，热毒血痢，风热感冒，温病发热。

（辛贵忠）

Experiment 4　The Determination of Chlorogenic Acid in Lonicerae Japonicae Flos by HPLC

Purpose

1. Comprehend the properties of chlorogenic acid and its quantitative methods.

2. Comprehend the application of high performance liquid chromatography in the determination of organic acids.

Principles

Lonicerae Japonicae Flos is a commonly used Chinese herb with multiple actions. It contains many kinds of substances, such as organic acid, iridoids and flavonoids. Among them, chlorogenic acid plays a very important role in quality control for this drug. The Chinese Pharmacopoeia recorded that the total content of chlorogenic acid in Lonicerae Japonicae Flos should be not less than 1.5%. In this experiment, HPLC method will be employed in the assay of Lonicerae Japonicae Flos.

Conditions

1. Apparatus　HPLC instrument, C_{18} column, ultrasonic cleaner, etc..

2. Reagents and materials　Lonicerae Japonicae Flos, chlorogenic acid CRS, acetonitrile, methanol and water.

Experimental Procedure

1. Chromatographic system and system suitability　Use octadecylsilane bonded silica gel as the stationary phase and a mixture of acetonitrile and 0.4% phosphoric acid solution (13∶87) as the mobile phase, the wavelength of the detector is 327nm. The number of the oretical plates of the column is not less than 1000, calculated with reference to the peak of chlorogenic acid.

2. Reference solution Weigh accurately 2.0mg of chlorogenic acid CRS and dissolve in 2ml of 50% methanol, mix well as the standard stock solution. Measure accurately different volumes of the stock solution, respectively, into a volumetric flask and dilute with 50% methanol to produce a series of solutions containing 20、40、60、200、400μg of chlorogenic acid per ml.

3. Test solution Weigh accurately 0.5g of the sample powder (through No. 4 sieve) to a 100ml conical flask, add 50ml of 50% methanol and weigh. Ultrasonicate for 30 minutes (power, 250W; frequency, 35kHz) and weigh again, replenish the loss of solvent with 50% methanol, filter. Transfer accurately 5ml of the successive filtrate to a 25ml volumetric flask and dilute with 50% methanol to volume. Filter through a 0.45μm millipore memberine and use the successive filtrate as the test solution.

Procedure

Accurately inject 10μl of each of the reference solution and the test solution respectively into the column, determine and calculate the content.

Experiment records

1. Record the results of this experiment, and plot the standard curve and calculate the regression equation and correlation coefficient.

2. Calculate the content ofchlorogenic acid in Lonicerae Japonicae Flos.

Questions

What other methods are used for determining organic acids?

Background Information

1. Origins Lonicerae Japonicae Flos is the dried flower bud of *Lonicera japonica* Thumb. (Fam. Caprifoliaceae). The flower is collected before flowering in early summer and dried.

2. Chemical constituents Chlorogenic acid ($C_{16}H_{18}O_9$): The molecular weight is 354.31; the melting point is 207 ~ 209℃; It is insoluble in chloroform or other lipophilic solvents while it is soluble in ethanol and acetone.

Chlorogenic acid is a natural chemical compound which is the ester of caffeic acid and (−) −quinic acid. Chlorogenic acid is an important intermediate in lignin biosynthesis. This compound, known as an antioxidant, may also slow the release of glucose into the blood after a meal.

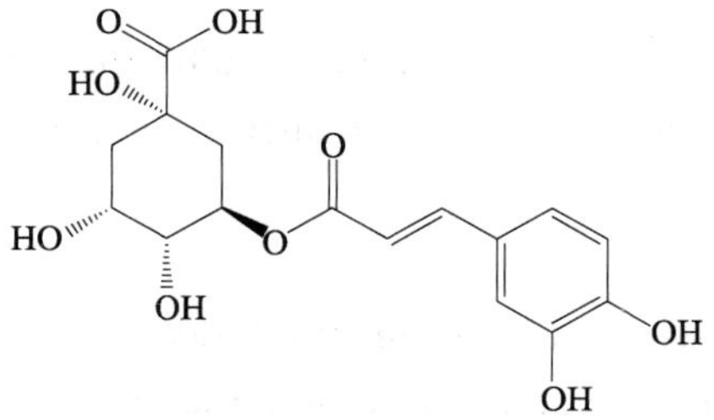

chlorogenic acid

3. Actions and indications To clear *heat* and remove toxin, disperse wind – heat. Used for swelling abscess, deep – rooted boil and sore, throat impediment, erysipelas, heat – toxin blood dysentery, common cold caused by wind – heat, fever in warm disease.

(Guizhong Xin)

第七章
中药制剂质量分析

实验一　双黄连口服液的质量分析

【实验目的】

1. 熟悉黄酮类化合物的性质。

2. 了解中药口服液制剂分析的一般方法。

【实验原理】

双黄连口服液由黄芩、金银花、连翘三味中药组成，黄芩苷是其主要有效成分之一，本实验选择高效液相色谱法，通过测定黄芩苷的含量对双黄连口服液进行质量控制。

【实验器材】

1. 仪器　高效液相色谱仪，ODS 色谱柱，电子分析天平，超声波清洗器，聚酰胺薄膜，量瓶，三用紫外分析仪。

2. 试药与试剂　双黄连口服液，黄芩苷，乙醇，甲醇，醋酸。

【实验步骤】

1. 定性分析　取本品 1ml，加 75% 乙醇 5ml，摇匀，作为供试品溶液。另取黄芩苷对照品，加 75% 的乙醇制成每 1ml 含 0.1mg 的溶液，作为对照品溶液。照薄层色谱法试验，吸取上述两种溶液各 2μl，分别点于同一聚酰胺薄膜上，以醋酸为展开剂，展开，取出，晾干，置紫外灯 365nm 下检视。供试品色谱中，在与对照品色谱相应的位置上，显相同的红色斑点。

2. 定量分析

（1）色谱条件　以十八烷基键合硅胶为固定相，以甲醇 – 水 – 冰醋酸（50∶50∶1）为流动相，检测波长 274nm。

（2）对照品溶液的制备　取黄芩苷对照品适量，精密称定，加 50% 甲醇制成每 1ml 含 0.1mg 的溶液，即得。

（3）供试品溶液的制备　精密量取本品 1ml，置 50ml 量瓶中，加 50% 甲醇适量，超声处理 20 分钟，放冷至室温，加 50% 甲醇稀释至刻度，摇匀，即得。

（4）测定法　分别精密吸取对照品溶液与供试品溶液各 5μl，注入液相色谱仪，测定，即得。

【实验记录】

1. 绘制定性鉴别色谱图，计算黄芩苷的 R_f值。

2. 计算双黄连口服液中黄芩苷的百分含量。

【思考题】

1. 进行定量分析时，口服制剂常用的预处理方法有哪些？

2. 如何制备双黄连口服液的阴性对照溶液？

【相关资料】

1. 药材来源　双黄连口服液由黄芩、金银花、连翘三味中药组成。

2. 主要化学成分　双黄连口服液主要含有黄芩苷、汉黄芩苷、黄芩素、绿原酸、连翘苷、连翘酚等。黄芩苷为黄色针状结晶，分子量 446.36，分子式 $C_{21}H_{18}O_{11}$，熔点 223 ~ 225℃。

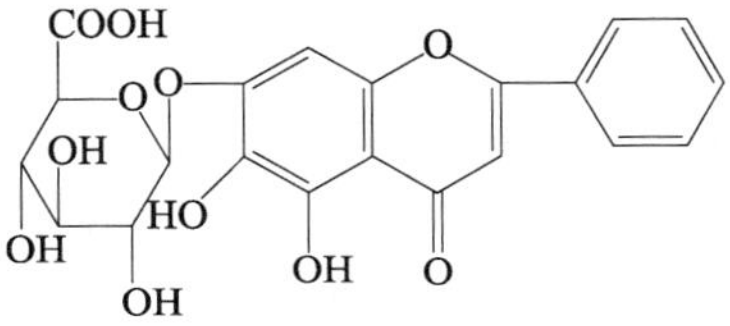

黄芩苷

3. 功能与主治　疏风解表，清热解毒。用于外感风热所致的感冒，症见发热、咳嗽、咽痛。

Experiment 1　The Quality Analysis of Shuanghuanglian Mixture

Purpose

1. Understand the properties of flavonoids.

2. Know about the common methods to assay the oral liquid in Chinese medicine preparations.

Principle

Shuanghuanglian Mixture is composed of Scutellaria Radix, Lonicerae Japonicae Flos and Forsythiae Fructus. Baicalin is the main active ingredient. In this experiment, HPLC method was carried out in determination of baicalin in sample for the quality control on this preparation.

Conditions

1. Apparatus　HPLC instrument, ODS column, electronic analytical balance, ultrasonic cleaner, polyamide membrane, volumetric flask and ultraviolet analyzer.

2. Reagents and materials　Shuanghuanglian Mixture, baicalin CRS, acetic acid, ethanol and methanol.

Experimental Procedure

1. Qualitative analysis Mix well 1ml of the sample with 5ml of 75% ethanol as the test solution. Dissolve baicalin CRS in 75% ethanol to produce a solution containing 0. 1mg per ml as the reference solution. Carry out the method for thin layer chromatography, using polyamide membrane as the coating substance and acetic acid as the mobile phase. Apply separately 2μl of each of the above two solutions to membrane. After developing and removal of the membrane, dry in air, examine under ultraviolet light at 365nm. The fluorescence spot and spot in the chromatogram obtained with the reference solution correspond in position and colour to the spot in the chromatogram obtained with the baicalin reference solution.

2. Quantitative analysis

(1) Chromatograhic system Use octadecylsilane bonded silica gel as the stationary phase and a mixture of methanol, water and glacial acetic acid (50∶50∶1) as the mobile phase. The wave length of detection is 274nm.

(2) Reference solution Weigh accurately a quantity of baicalin CRS, dissolve in 50% methanol to produce a solution containing 0. 1mg per ml as the reference solution.

(3) Test solution Measure accurately 1ml of the mixture into a 50ml volumetric flask, add a quantity of 50% methanol, ultrasonicate for 20 minutes, stand to room temperature, dilute with 50% methanol to volume and mix well.

(4) Procedure Inject accurately 5μl of each of the reference solution and the test solution into the column and calculate the content.

Experiment records

1. Draw the thin layer chromatogram of identification and calculate R_f value of main spots.

2. Calculate the content (%) of baicalin in Shuanghuanglian Mixture.

Qusetions

1. What are the commonly used methods of pretreatments of oral preparations in the quantitative analysis?

2. How to prepare the negative control solution of Shuanghuanglian Koufuye?

Background Information

1. Origins Shuanghuanglian Mixture is composed of Scutellaria Radix, Lonicerae Japonicae Flos and Forsythiae Fructus.

2. Chemical constituents The drug mainly contains baicalin, wogonoside, chlorogenic acid, forsythin, forsythol and so on. Baicalin is yellow needle crystal. The molecular weight is 446. 36. The molecular formula is $C_{21}H_{18}O_{11}$. Melting point is 223 ~ 225℃.

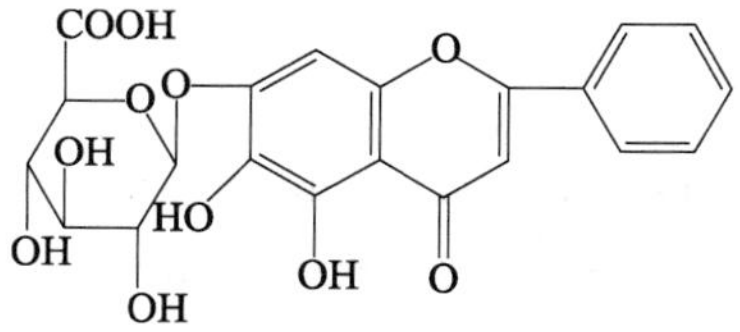

baicalin

3. Actions and indications　To disperse *wind*, release the exterior pattern, clear heat and remove toxin. Cold caused by externally contracted wind – heat manifested as fever, cough, and painful throat.

实验二　元胡止痛片的质量分析

【实验目的】

1. 掌握薄层层析法在中药制剂定性分析中的应用。
2. 熟悉含生物碱类成分中药制剂的一般精制方法。

【实验原理】

元胡止痛片由延胡索、白芷两味药材组成，其中生物碱是延胡索中的主要活性成分，本实验根据甲基橙与延胡素总生物碱生成稳定的有色离子对化合物，用三氯甲烷提取后，采用比色法测定该片剂中延胡素总生物碱的含量。

【实验器材】

1. 仪器　电子天平，超声仪，可见 – 紫外分光光度计，硅胶 G 薄层板，毛细管，容量瓶。

2. 试药与试剂　元胡止痛片，延胡索乙素，氧化铝，氨水，乙醚，甲醇，1% 氢氧化钠，正已烷，三氯甲烷，0.1mol/L 盐酸，碘蒸气，醋酸 – 醋酸钠缓冲液（pH 4.5）：取醋酸钠 18g，加冰醋酸 9.8ml，再加水稀释至 1000ml；0.2% 甲基橙水溶液。

【实验步骤】

1. 定性分析　取本品 10 片，除去包衣，研细，加甲醇 50ml，超声处理 30min，滤过，滤液加活性氧化铝 5g，振摇数分钟，滤过，滤液蒸干，残渣加水适量使溶解，加浓氨试液调 pH 值至碱性，用乙醚振摇提取 3 次，每次 10ml，乙醚液蒸干，残渣加甲醇 1ml 使溶解，作为供试品溶液。另取延胡索乙素对照品适量，制成每 1ml 含 0.1mg 的溶液，作为对照品溶液。照薄层色谱法试验，吸取上述两种溶液各 2 ~ 3μl，分别点于同一用 1% 氢氧化钠溶液制备的硅胶 G 薄层板上，以正已烷 – 三氯甲烷 – 甲醇（7.5∶4∶1）为展开剂，展开，取出，晾干，以碘蒸气熏至斑点显色。

2. 定量分析

（1）对照品溶液的制备　精密称取延胡索乙素对照品适量，用 0.1mol/L HCl 溶液溶解制成，每 1ml 含延胡索乙素 0.156mg。

（2）样品溶液的制备　取元胡止痛片 10 片，除去糖衣，研细，取细粉约 0.3g，精密称定，置 50ml 量瓶中，加 0.1mol/L HCl 溶液约 40ml，水浴加热 20 分钟，时时振摇，取出放冷，加同一溶液至刻度，摇匀，过滤，弃去初滤液，留取续滤液，备用。

（3）标准曲线的制备　精密吸取对照品溶液 0、0.2、0.4、0.6、0.8、1.0ml，分别置于分液漏斗中，各加醋酸 – 醋酸钠缓冲液 10.0ml，0.2% 甲基橙溶液 1.0ml，再加入三氯甲烷 10ml，振摇 3 分钟，静置使分层，分取三氯甲烷液，精密吸取三氯甲烷液 1ml。以第一管为空白，在 420nm 波长处测定吸收度，将测定的数据进行线性回归计算。

（4）样品的测定　吸取样品溶液 1ml，置于分液漏斗中，各加醋酸 – 醋酸钠缓冲液

10.0ml，0.2%甲基橙溶液1.0ml，再加入三氯甲烷10ml，振摇3分钟，静置使分层，分取三氯甲烷液，精密吸取样品液1ml，在420nm波长处测定吸收度。

【实验记录】

1. 简述操作过程，记录实验现象。
2. 绘制定性层析图谱，计算 R_f 值。
3. 计算元胡止痛片中总生物碱的含量。

【思考题】

1. 定性鉴别实验时，供试品溶液的制备中各步骤的操作目的是什么？
2. 简述本实验中定量分析方法的优点和不足，请设计其他定量分析实验方法。

【相关资料】

1. 药材来源 元胡止痛片由延胡索、白芷两味中药组成。

2. 主要化学成分 元胡止痛片主要含延胡素甲素、乙素、丙素、丁素、欧前胡素、异欧前胡素、比克白芷素等。延胡素乙素为白色结晶，分子量355.42，分子式 $C_{21}H_{25}NO_4$，熔点148～149℃，易溶于乙醚和三氯甲烷，不溶于水。

3. 功能与主治 理气、活血、止痛。用于气滞血瘀的胃痛、胁痛、头痛及痛经。

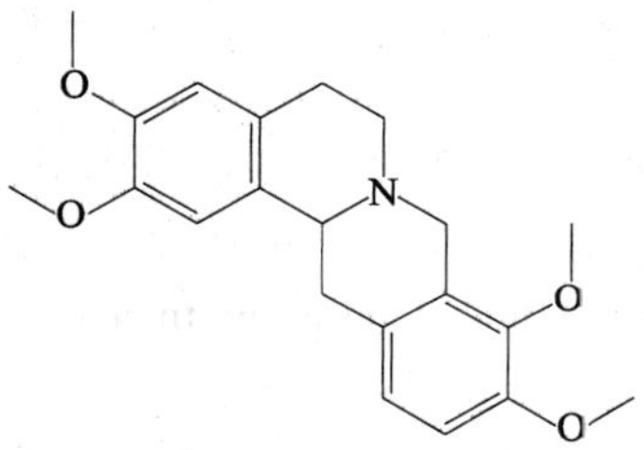

延胡素乙素

Experiment 2 The Quality Analysis of Yuanhu Zhitong Tablets

Purpose

1. Comprehend the application of thin – layer chromatogram in analysis of Chinese medicine preparations.

2. Understand the extraction method of Chinese medicine preparations containing alkaloids.

Principle

Tablets are composed of two kinds of crude drug, Corydalis Rhizoma and Angelicae Dahuricae Radix. Among them, alkaloids are major active ingredients in Rhizoma Corydalis. In this experiment, the content of total alkaloid in this compound tablets were determined by colorimetric method based on colored ion pair compounds produced from methyl orange and Yanhusuo total alkaloids.

Conditions

1. Apparatus Electronic balance, ultrasonic cleaner, UV – VIS spectrophotometer, silica gel G plate, capillary tube and volumetric flask.

2. Reagents and materials Yuanhu Zhitong Tablets, terahydropalmatine, alumina, ammonia, ether, methanol, 1% solution of sodium hydroxide, *n* – hexane, chloroform, 0. 1% hydrochloric acid solution, iodine vapor, acetic acid – sodium acetate (pH 4. 5): weigh accurately 18g of glacial acetic acid, then dilute to 1000ml with water 0. 2% methyl orange solution.

Experimental Procedure

1. Qualitative analysis To 10 tablets, removed the coats, add 50ml of methanol, ultrasonicate for 30 minutes, and filter, add 5g of aluminium oxide activated to the filtrate, shake for several minutes, and filter. Evaporate the filtrate to dryness, dissolve the residue in water, alkalify with concentrated ammonia TS, and then extract with three 10ml quantities of ether with shaking. Combine the ether extracts and evaporate to dryness, dissolve the residue in 1ml of methanol as the test solution. Disslove a quantity of tetrahydropalmatine CRS, weigh accurately, in methanol to produce a solution containing 0. 1mg per ml as the reference solution. Carry out the method for thin layer chromatography, using silica gel G mixed with 1% solution of sodium hydroxide as the coating substance and a mixture of *n* – hexane, chloroform and methanol (7. 5: 4: 1) as the mobile phase. Apply separately 2 ~ 3μl of each of the two solutions to the plate. After developing in a chamber pre – equilibrated with the mobile phase for 1 hour and removal the plate, dry in air, expose the plate to iodine vapor until the spots clear.

2. Quantitative analysis

(1) Reference solution Disslove a quantity of tetrahydropalmatine CRS, accurately weighed, in 0. 1mol/L hydrochloric acid to produce a solution containing 0. 156mg per ml as the reference solution.

(2) Test solution Take 10 tabltes, remove coats and accurately weigh, pulverize to fine powder, weigh accurately 0. 3g to a 50ml volumetric flask, add 40ml of 0. 1mm hydrochloric acid solution, warm on a water bath for 20 mimutes with constantly shaking, take out and cool, dilute with 0. 1mm hydrochloric acid solution to volume, mix well, filter, discard the initial filtrate, use the successive filtrate as the test solution.

(3) Preparation of standard curve Transfer accurately 0, 0. 2, 0. 4, 0. 6, 0. 8 and 1. 0ml of reference solution to separating funnel, respectively, add 10ml of acetic acid – sodium acetate buffer, 1ml of 0. 2% methyl orange solution and 10ml of chloroform, and mix well, alow to stand and separate the chloroform layer. Transfer accurately 1ml of each of the chloroform solutions to volumetric flask. Use the first solution as a blank, measure the absorbance at 420nm and plot the standard curve.

(4) Assay Transfer accurately 1ml of the test solution to separating funnel, add 10ml acetic acid – sodium acetate of buffer, 1ml of 0. 2% methyl orange solution and 10ml of

chloroform, mix well, allow to stand, separate the chloroform layer. Transfer accurately 1ml of the chloroform solution to volumetric flask. Measure the absorbance at 420nm and calculate the content according to the standard curve.

Experiment records

1. Describe the process of this experiment briefly, and record the test phenomena.

2. Draw the qualitative thin layer chromatogram, and calculate the R_f value of major spots.

3. Calculate the content of total alkaloids in Yuanhu Zhitong Tabltes.

Questions

1. What is purpose of each procedure of preparation of test solution in qualitative analysis?

2. Draw the advantages and disadvantages of the quantitative method and design other method to determine the content.

Background Information

1. Origins Yuanhu Zhitong Tablets are composed of two kinds of crude drug, Corydalis Rhizoma and *Angelicae Dahuricae* Radix.

2. Chemical constituents Yuanhu Zhitong Tablets contain *d* – corydaline, *dl* – tetrahydropaimatine, protopine, *l* – tetrahydro coptisine, Imperatorin, Isoimperatorin, byakangelicin. Terahydropalmatine is a white crystal, its molecular weight is 355.42. The molecular formula is $C_{21}H_{25}NO_4$, The mp is between 148 ~ 149℃. It can be highly disslove in ether or chloroform and almost insoluble in water.

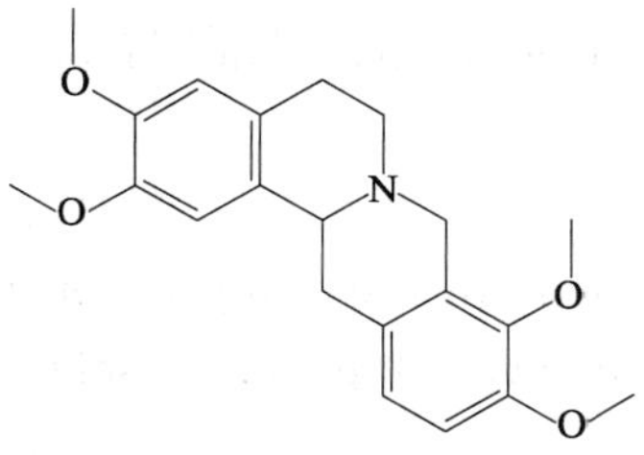

terahydropalmatine

3. Actions and indications To regulate *qi*, activate blood, and relieve pain. Used for stomachache, hypochondriac pain, headache, dysmenorrhea caused by *qi* stagnation and blood stasis.

实验三　六味地黄丸的质量分析

【实验目的】

1. 掌握高效液相色谱法在中药制剂定量分析中的应用。

2. 熟悉丸剂常规预处理方法。

【实验原理】

六味地黄丸由熟地黄、牡丹皮、山茱萸、山药、茯苓、泽泻等六味中药组成，其中丹皮酚是牡丹皮中的主要活性成分，在 274nm 处有最大吸收，故选用紫外检测器在 274nm 波长处进行测定。

【实验器材】

1. 仪器　高效液相色谱仪、硅胶 G 薄层板、ODS 柱、电子天平、具塞锥形瓶、超声波清洗仪。

2. 试药与试剂　丹皮酚对照品、六味地黄丸、硅藻土、甲醇、乙腈、水、乙醚、丙酮、环己烷、乙酸乙酯、酸性 5% 三氯化铁乙醇液。

【实验步骤】

1. 定性分析　取本品水蜜丸 6g，研细，加硅藻土 4g，研匀，加乙醚 40ml，回流 1 小时，滤过，滤液挥去乙醚，残渣加丙酮 1ml 使溶解，作为供试品溶液。另取丹皮酚对照品，加丙酮制成每 1ml 含 1mg 的溶液，作为对照品溶液。照薄层色谱法试验，吸取上述两种溶液各 10μl，分别点于同一硅胶 G 薄层板上，以环己烷－乙酸乙酯（3∶1）为展开剂，展开，取出，晾干，喷以酸性 5% 三氯化铁乙醇溶液，加热至斑点显色。

2. 定量分析

（1）色谱条件　色谱柱为 ODS 柱（250mm × 4.6mm，5μm），柱温为 35℃，检测波长为 274nm，流动相为甲醇－水（65∶35），流速为 1ml/min。

（2）对照品溶液的制备　精密称取丹皮酚对照品适量，加甲醇制成 25μg/ml 的溶液，即得。

（3）供试品溶液的制备　取本品研细，取 0.5g，精密称定，置于具塞锥形瓶中，精密加入甲醇 50ml，密塞，称定质量，超声处理 30 分钟，放冷，再称定质量，用甲醇补足减失的质量，摇匀，滤过，取续滤液，即得。

（4）测定法　取样品按定性分析项下供试品溶液的制备方法制得供试品溶液，进样测定，按外标法计算含量。

【实验记录】

1. 简述操作过程，记录实验现象。
2. 绘制定性层析图谱，计算 R_f 值。
3. 计算六味地黄丸中丹皮酚的含量。

【思考题】

1. 本实验中定性分析方法的缺点是什么？
2. 请设计用其他方法测定六味地黄丸中丹皮酚的含量。

【相关资料】

1. 药材来源　六味地黄丸由熟地黄、牡丹皮、山茱萸、山药、茯苓、泽泻等六味中药制成。

2. 主要化学成分　熟地黄主要含有梓醇、地黄苷、桃叶珊瑚苷、地黄素、单萜成分等。牡丹皮含有丹皮酚、丹皮酚苷、芍药苷、苯甲酰芍药苷等。山茱萸含有挥发油、鞣质、环烯醚萜类成分等。山药含有多糖、脂肪酸、酯类成分等。茯苓含有茯苓多糖、三萜类化合物等。泽泻含有泽泻醇等三萜类成分及倍半萜类、二萜类。丹皮酚为无色针状结晶（甲醇），分子量为 166.17，分子式 $C_9H_{10}O_3$，熔点 49～51℃。

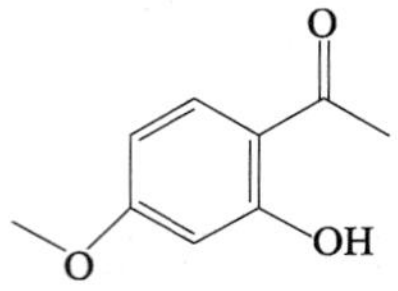

丹皮酚

3. 功能与主治 滋阴补肾。用于肾阴亏损，头晕耳鸣，腰膝酸软，骨蒸潮热，盗汗遗精，消渴。

Experiment 3 The Quality Analysis of Liuwei Dihuang Pills

Purpose

1. Comprehend the application of HPLC method in quantitative analysis of Chinese Medicine Preparations.

2. Understand the conventional pretreatment methods of pills.

Principle

Liuwei Dihuang Pills consist of six kinds of crude drugs. The ingredients are Rehmanniae Radix Praeparata, Corni Fructus, Moutan Cortex, Dioscoreae Rhizoma, Poria and Alismatis Rhizoma. Paeonol is the main component of cortex moutan, and has maximum absorption at 274nm. Hence, we choose ultraviolet detector at 274nm wavelengths to measure.

Conditions

1. Apparatus HPLC instrument, silica gel G plate, C_{18} column, electronic balance, stopper conical flask and ultrasonic cleaner.

2. Reagents and materials Paeonol CRS, Liuwei Dihuang Pills, kieselguhr, ethanol, acetonitrile, water, ethyl ether, acetone, cyclohexane, ethyl acetate and 5% acidic ferric chloride ethanol solution.

Experimental Procedure

1. Qualitative analysis Pulverize 6g of the water honeyed pills with 4g of kieselguhr and triturate well. Heat under reflux with 40ml of ether at a low temperature for 1 hour, filter and expel ether. Dissovle the residue in 1ml of acetone as the test solution. Dissolve paeonol CRS in acetone to preparea solution containing 1mg per ml as the reference solution. Carry out the method for thin layer chromatography, using silica gel G as the coating substance and cyclohexane and ethyl acetate (3∶1) as the mobile phase. Apply separately 10μl of each of the two solutions to the plate. After developing and removal of the plate, dry in air, spray with 5% ferric chloride in ethanol acidified with hydrochloric acid and heat to the spots clear. The bluish brown spot in the chromatogram obtained with the test solution corresponds in position and colour to the spot in the chromatogram obtained with the reference solution.

2. Quantitative analysis

(1) Chromatographic system Use octadecylsilane bonded silica gel as the stationary

phase (250mm × 4.6mm, 5μm) and a mixture of methanol and water (65∶35) as the mobile phase, flow rate: 1ml/min, The wavelength of the detection is 274nm and the column temperature is set at 35℃.

(2) Reference solution　Dissolve a quantity of paeonol CRS, accurately weighed, in 50% methanol to prepare a solution containing 25μg per ml.

(3) Test solution　Pulverize a quantity of water – honeyed pills, weigh accurately 0.5g of the fine powder to a stopper conical flask, add accurately 50ml of 50% methanol, stopper tightly and weigh. Ultrasonicate for 30 minutes, cool and weigh again. Replenish the loss of solvent with 50% methanol, mix well and filter and use the successive filtrate as the test solution.

(4) Procedure　Inject accurately 10μl of each of the reference solution and the test solution into the column, determine and calculate the content.

Experiment records

1. Describe briefly the processes of the experiment.

2. Plot the TLC chromatogram for qualitative identification and calculate the R_f value of main spots.

3. Calculate the content of paeonol in sample.

Questions

1. What are the disadvantages of qualitative analysis of the experiment?

2. Please design another method to determinethe content of paeonol in sample.

Background Information

1. Origins　Liuwei Dihuang Pills consist of six kinds of crude drugs. The ingredients are Rehmanniae Radix Praeparata, Corni Fructus, Moutan Cortex, Dioscoreae Rhizoma, Poria and Alismatis Rhizoma.

2. Chemical constituents　Radix Rehmanniae praeparata mainly contain scatalpol, rehmannioside, aucubin, rehmannin, monoterpene and so on. The contents of Cortex Moutan are paeonol, paeonoside, paeoniflorin, benzoyl paeoniflorin, etc. Fructus Corni contains volatile oils, tannins, cycloalkene ether terpenoids composition, etc. Rhizoma Dioscoreae consists of polysaccharides, fatty acids, esters, etc. Poria contains pachman and triterpenoid etc. Rhizoma Alismatis consists of alisol, sesquiterpenoids, diterpenes and so on. Paeonol is colorless needle crystal (ethanol), the molecular weight: 166.17, molecular formula: $C_9H_{10}O_3$, melting point: 49 ~ 51℃.

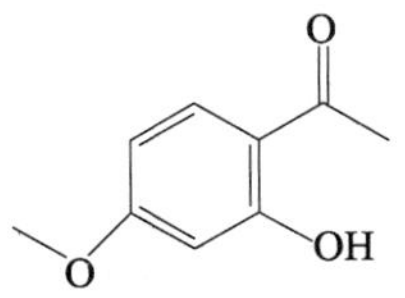

paeonol

3. Actions and indications　To nourish *yin* to tonify the kidney. Kidney *yin* deficiency pattern manifested as dizziness, tinnitus, soreness and weakness in the lower back and knees, bone－steaming with tidal fever, night sweating, seminal emission and consumptive thirst.

实验四　复方丹参滴丸的质量分析

【实验目的】

1. 掌握内标法测定样品含量的计算。

2. 熟悉气相色谱仪的原理及使用。

【实验原理】

复方丹参滴丸由丹参、三七、冰片组成，本实验利用正丁烷萃取冰片成分，加入一定量的内标物质，用气相色谱法进行定量分析。

【实验器材】

1. 仪器　气相色谱仪，石英毛细管柱，超声仪，硅胶 G 薄层板。

2. 试药与试剂　复方丹参滴丸，冰片，无水乙醇，环己烷，乙酸乙酯，1% 香草醛硫酸，正己烷，正丁烷。

3. 内标物：萘。

【实验步骤】

1. 定性分析　取本品 40 丸，研碎，加无水乙醇 10ml，超声处理 10 分钟，滤过，滤液作为供试品溶液。另取冰片对照品，加无水乙醇制成每 1ml 含 1mg 的溶液，作为对照品溶液。照薄层色谱法试验，吸取上述两种溶液各 5～10μl，分别点于同一硅胶 G 薄层板上，以环己烷－乙酸乙酯（17∶3）为展开剂，展开，取开，晾干，喷以 1% 香草醛硫酸溶液，在 105℃加热显色。

2. 定量分析

（1）色谱条件与系统适用性试验　石英毛细管柱，以交联苯甲基聚硅氧烷作为固定液，涂布浓度为 5%；FID 检测器，检测器温度 200℃；气化室温度 200℃；氮气为载气，载气流速 1.0ml/min；柱温度以 60℃为初始温度，以 20℃每分钟的速度升温至 150℃，维持 4min。理论板数按龙脑峰计算，应不低于 2000。

（2）内标液的配制　精确称取 0.160g 萘置于 100ml 量瓶中，加正己烷稀释至刻度，浓度为 1.6mg/ml。

（3）对照品溶液的配制　精确称取龙脑 50mg，置于 25ml 棕色量瓶中，加上述内标液溶解并稀释至刻度，摇匀，即得，龙脑含量为 2mg/ml。

（4）样品溶液的制备　取本品滴丸 20 丸，精确称定，加 5ml 蒸馏水，完全溶解后，用正丁烷萃取 3 次（10ml、5ml、5ml），萃取液置于 25ml 量瓶中，精取内标液 1ml 置于同一量瓶中，用正己烷溶解并稀释至刻度，摇匀，即得。

（5）线性关系考察　精确称取龙脑对照品 25mg 置于 25ml 量瓶中，加正己烷稀释至刻度。分别精确量取该溶液 0.5、1.0、1.5、2.0、3.0ml，置于 5ml 量瓶中，用内标液定容至刻度，摇匀待测，分别进行 2μl 按前述色谱条件测定峰面积，以龙脑峰为纵坐标，龙脑浓度（mg/ml）为横坐标，进行线性回归。

（6）测定法　吸取样品溶液 2μl 注入气相色谱仪，测定，即得。

【实验记录】

1. 画出定性薄层图，计算冰片的 R_f 值。
2. 计算复方丹参滴丸中冰片的含量。

【思考题】

1. 用气相色谱法测定中药制剂中的有效成分需注意哪些问题？
2. 采用内标法计算含量的优点是什么？

【相关资料】

1. 药材来源　复方丹参滴丸由丹参、三七、冰片组成。

2. 主要化学成分　复方丹参滴丸主要含有丹参素、原儿茶醛、丹酚酸、丹参酮、三七皂苷、人参皂苷、冰片等。冰片又名龙脑，白色、半透明结晶，分子量 154.25，分子式 $C_{10}H_{18}O$，熔点 208℃，不溶于水，溶于乙醇、三氯甲烷、乙醚。具有类似樟脑的气味。

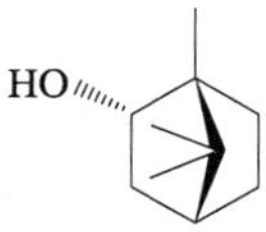

龙脑

3. 功能与主治　活血化瘀，理气止痛。用于气滞血瘀所致的胸痹，症见胸闷、心前区刺痛，冠心病心绞痛见上述症状者。

（夏玉凤）

Experiment 4　The Quality Analysis of Compound Danshen Dripping Pills

Purpose

1. Comprehend the operation of the gas chromatography.
2. Master the calculation of percentage content of the sample by internal standard method.

Principle

Compound Danshen Dripping Pills are made up of Salvia Miltiorrhizae Radix et Rhizoma, Notoginseng Radix et Rhizoma, and Borneolum Syntheticum. Extract the borneol with *n* – butane, add a quality of internal standard substance, and then determine by gas chromatography.

Conditions

1. Apparatus　Gas chromatograph, quartz capillary column, ultrasonic cleaner and silica gel G plate.

2. Reagents and materials　Compound Danshen Dripping Pills, borneol CRS, naphthalene, dehydrated ethanol, eyclohexane, ethyl acetate, 1% vanillin sulfuric acid, n – hexane and *n* – butane.

3. Internal standard naphthalene.

Experimental Procedure

1. Qualitative analysis Pulverize 40 pills to powder, add 10ml of dehydrated ethanol. Ultrasonicate for 10 minutes, filter, and use the filtrate as the test solution. Dissolve borneol CRS in dehydrated ethanol to prepare a solution containing 1mg per ml as the reference solution. Carry out the method for thin layer chromatography, using silica gel G as the coating substance and a mixture of cyclohexane and ethyl acetate (17 : 3) as the mobile phase. Apply separately 5 ~ 10μl of each of the two solutions to the plate. After developing and removal of the plate, dry in air, spray with 1% solution of vanillin in sulfuric acid, heat at 105℃ to the spots clear. The spot in the chromatogram obtained with the test solution corresponds in position and colour to the spot in the chromatogram obtained with the reference solution.

2. Quantitative analysis

(1) Chromatographic system and system suitability Quartz capillary column, crosslinked styrene methyl polysiloxane as the stationary liquid, and coating concentration is 5%. Detector temperature is set at 200℃ and the vaporizing chamber temperature is 200℃. The flow rate of carrier gas (N_2) is 1. 0ml/min.

The program temperature: the initial column temperature is 60℃ and increase to 150℃ at a rate of 20℃ per minute and maintain 4 minutes.

The number of theoretical plates of the column is not less than 2000, calculated with reference to the peak of borneol.

(2) Internal standard solution Dissolve 0. 160g of naphthalene, accurately weighed, in a 100ml volumetric flask, dilute with *n* – hexane to volume to prepare a solution containing 1. 6mg per ml.

(3) Reference solution Weigh accurately 50mg of borneol, into a brown 25ml volumetric flask, add internal standard solution, and swirl until dissolved. Dilute with internal standard solution to volume, and mix, contain borneol 2mg per ml.

(4) Test solution Weigh accurately 20 pills of Compound Danshen Dripping Pills, dissolved in 5ml of distilled water and swirl until dissolved, extracted with *n* – butane for 3 times (10ml, 5ml, 5ml), Combine the extracts to a 25ml volumetric flask, add internal standard solution, and mix well. Dilute with *n* – hexane to volume, and mix well as the test solution.

(5) Standard curve Weigh accurately 25mg of borneol CRS, in a 25ml volumetric flask. Dissolve with *n* – hexane to volume, and mix well. Transfer accurately 0. 5ml, 1. 0ml, 1. 5ml, 2. 0ml, 3. 0ml of the solution, respectively, into a 5ml volumetric flask. Dilute with internal standard solution to volume, and shake well. Inject 2μl of the above five solutions respectively under the same chromatographic system to determine peak area. Draw the standard curve with peak area as the ordinate and the concentration (mg/ml) as the abscissa.

(6) Procedure　Inject 2μl of test solution under the same chromatographic system and calculate the content.

Experiment records

1. Plot the TLC for qualitative identification and calculate the R_f value.

2. Calculate the content of borneol in complex salvia miltiorrhiza drill.

Questions

1. What should we pay more attention to in using gas chromatography to determine the effective constituent of traditional Chinese preparations.

2. What are the advantages of using internal standard method to calculate the content?

Background Information

1. Origins　Danshen Dripping Pills is made up of *Salvia Miltiorrhizae* Radix et Rhizoma, Notoginseng Radix et Rhizoma, and Borneolum Syntheticum.

2. Chemical constituents　Danshen Dropping Pill mostly contains, tanshinol, protocatechuic aldehyde, phenolic acids, tanshinone, panax notoginseng saponins, ginseng saponin, borneol and so on. Borneol is white and translucent crystal, with volatile, molecular weight: 154.25, molecular formula: $C_{10}H_{18}O$, melting point: 208℃, Borneol is insoluble in water, soluble in ethanol, chloroform, ethyl ether, similar to the smell of camphor.

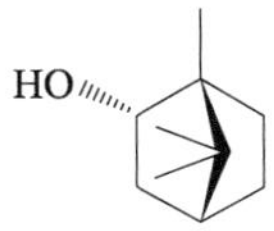

borneol

3. Actions and indications　To promote blood circulation, to resolve stagnated blood and regulate *qi* flow to kill pain. Impeded flow of *yang qi* in the chest due to stagnation of *qi* and blood with manifestations of constriction and stabbing pain in the precardium, angina pectoris in coronary heart disease with above symptoms.

(Yufeng Xia)

附录

附录一　常用中药质量分析方法

一、分光光度法

分光光度法是通过测定被测物质在特定波长处或一定波长范围内的光吸收度，对该物质进行定性和定量分析的方法。

常用的波长范围为：①200～400nm 的紫外光区；②400～760nm 的可见光区；③2.5～25μm（按波数计为 4000～400cm^{-1}）的红外光区。所用仪器为紫外分光光度计、可见分光光度计（或比色计）、红外分光光度计或原子吸收分光光度计。为保证测量的精密度和准确度，所有仪器应按照国家计量检定规程或本附录规定，定期进行校正检定。

单色光辐射穿过被测物质溶液时，被该物质吸收的量与该物质的浓度和液层的厚度（光路长度）成正比，其关系如下式：

$$A = \lg \frac{1}{T} = ECL$$

式中　A 为吸收度；

T 为透光率；

E 为吸收系数，采用的表示方法是（$E_{1cm}^{1\%}$），其物理意义为当溶液浓度为 1%（g/ml），液层厚度为 1cm 时的吸收度数值；

C 为 100ml 溶液中所含被测物质的重量（按干燥品或无水物计算），g；

L 为液层厚度，cm。

物质对光的选择性吸收波长，以及相应的吸收系数是该物质的物理常数。当已知某纯物质在一定条件下的吸收系数后，可用同样条件将该供试品配成溶液，测定其吸收度，即可由上式计算出供试品中该物质的含量。在可见光区，除某些物质对光有吸收外，很多物质本身并没有吸收，但可在一定条件下加入显色试剂或经过处理使其显色后再测定，故又称比色分析。由于显色时影响呈色深浅的因素较多，且常使用单色光纯度较差的仪器，故测定时应用标准品或对照品同时操作。

二、紫外分光光度法

1. 仪器的校正和检定　由于温度变化对机械部分的影响，仪器的波长经常会略有变动，因此除应定期对所用的仪器进行全面校正检定外，还应于测定前校正测定波长。常用汞灯中的较强谱线 237.83nm、253.65nm、275.28nm、296.73nm、313.16nm、334.15nm、365.02nm、404.66nm、435.83nm、546.07nm 与 576.96nm，或用仪器中氘灯的486.02nm与656.10nm谱线进行校正，钬玻璃在279.4nm、287.5nm、333.7nm、360.9nm、418.5nm、460.0nm、484.5nm、536.2nm与637.5nm波长处有尖锐吸收峰，也可作波长校正用，但因来源不同会有微小的差别，使用时应注意。

表附1-1 重铬酸钾的硫酸溶液吸收度表

波长/nm	235 (min)	257 (max)	313 (min)	350 (max)
吸收系数	124.5	144.0	48.62	106.6

吸收度的准确度可用重铬酸钾的硫酸溶液检定。取在120℃干燥至恒重的基准重铬酸钾约60mg，精密称定，用0.005mol/L硫酸溶液溶解并稀释至1000ml，在规定的波长处测定并计算其吸收系数，并与规定的吸收系数比较，如上表，相对偏差在±1%以内。

杂散光的检查可按下表的试剂和浓度，配制成水溶液，置1cm石英吸收池中，在规定的波长处测定透光率，应符合表中的规定。

表附1-2 杂散光检查限度

试剂	浓度% (g/ml)	测定用波长 (nm)	透光率%
碘化钠	1.00	220	<0.8
亚硝酸钠	5.00	340	<0.8

2. 对溶剂的要求 测定供试品前，应先检查所用的溶剂在供试品所用的波长附近是否符合要求，即用1cm石英吸收池盛溶剂，以空气为空白（即空白光路中不置任何物质）测定其吸收度。溶剂和吸收池的吸收度，在220~240nm范围内不得超过0.40，在241~250nm范围内不得超过0.20，在251~300nm范围内不得超过0.10，在300nm以上时不得超过0.05。

3. 测定法 测定时，除另有规定外，应以配制供试品溶液的同批溶剂为空白对照，采用1cm的石英吸收池，在规定的吸收峰波长±2nm以内测试几个点的吸收度，以核对供试品的吸收峰波长位置是否正确，除另有规定外，吸收峰波长应在该品种项下规定的波长±2nm以内；否则应考虑该试样的真伪、纯度以及仪器波长的准确度，并以吸收度最大的波长作为测定波长。一般供试品溶液的吸收度读数，以在0.3~0.7之间的误差较小。仪器的狭缝波带宽度应小于供试品吸收带的半宽度，否则测得的吸收度会偏低；狭缝宽度的选择，应以减小狭缝宽度时供试品的吸收度不再增加为准，由于吸收池和溶剂本身可能有空白吸收，因此测定供试品的吸收度后应减去空白读数，再计算含量。

用作鉴别和检查项目的方法，分别按各品种项下的方法进行。鉴别项下吸收度读数的范围可根据制剂的实际含量和供试液的稀释倍数估算。

用于含量测定的方法目前常用对照品比较法：

即按各品种项下的方法，分别配制供试品溶液和对照品溶液，对照品溶液中所含被测成分的量应为供试品溶液中被测成分标示量的100%±10%，所用溶剂也应完全一致，在规定的波长测定供试品溶液和对照品溶液的吸收度后，按下式计算供试品中被测溶液的浓度：

$$C_X = \frac{A_X}{A_R} C_R$$

式中　C_X为供试品溶液的浓度；
A_X为供试品溶液的吸收度；
C_R为对照品溶液的浓度；
A_R为对照品溶液的吸收度。

三、比色法

用比色法测定时，应取对照品同时操作。除另有规定外，比色法所用的空白系指用同体积的溶剂代替对照品或供试品溶液，然后依次加入等量的相应试剂，并用同样方法处理。在规定的波长处测定对照品和供试品溶液的吸收度后，按紫外分光光度法对照品比较法的计算式计算供试品浓度。

当吸收度和浓度关系不呈线形时，应取数份梯度量的对照品溶液，用溶剂补充至同一体积，显色后测定各份溶液的吸收度，然后以吸收度与相应的浓度绘制标准曲线，再根据供试品的吸收度在标准曲线上求出其含量。

四、原子吸收分光光度法

由待测元素灯发出的特征谱线通过供试品蒸汽时，被蒸汽中待测元素的基态原子所吸收，吸收遵循一般分光光度法的吸收定律，通过测定辐射光强度减弱的程度可求出供试品中待测元素的含量。通常借比较标准品和供试品的吸收度，求得供试品中待测元素的含量。

原子吸收分光光度法所用仪器为原子吸收分光光度计，它由光源、原子化器、单色器和检测器等部件组成。光源通常用待测元素作为阴极的空心阴极灯，原子化器由雾化器及燃烧灯头组成。燃烧火焰由不同种类的气体混合物产生，常用空气－乙炔火焰。仪器某些工作条件（如波长、狭缝、光源灯电流、火焰类型、火焰状态）的变化可影响灵敏度、稳定程度和干扰情况，应按各品种项下的规定选择。

1. 含量测定法

（1）第一法（标准曲线法）　在仪器推荐的浓度范围内，制备含待测元素的标准溶液至少 3 份，浓度依次递增，并分别加入供试品溶液配制中的相应试剂。除另有规定外，一般用去离子水制成水溶液。将仪器按规定启动后，先将去离子水喷入火焰，调读数为零，再将最浓的标准溶液喷入火焰，调节仪器至近满量程的读数；然后依次喷入每一标准溶液，读数。每喷完 1 份溶液后，均用去离子水喷入火焰充分冲洗灯头并调零。取每一浓度 3 次读数的平均值，与相应浓度作标准曲线。

按各品种项下的规定制备供试品溶液，使待测元素的估计浓度在标准曲线浓度范围内，将供试品溶液喷入火焰，取 3 次读数的平均值，从标准曲线上查得相应的浓度，计算元素的含量。

（2）第二法（标准加入法）　取同体积按各品种项下规定制备的供试品溶液 4 份，分别加至 4 个同体积的量瓶中，除①号量瓶外，其他②、③、④号量瓶分别再准确加入比例量的待测元素标准液，均用去离子水稀释至刻度，形成标准液加入量从零开始递增的一系列溶液。按上述标准曲线法自“将仪器按规定启动后”操作，并依次将溶液喷入火焰，读数；将读数与相应的待测元素加入量作图，延长此直线至与含量轴的延长线相交，此交点与原点间的距离即相当于供试品溶液取用量中待测元素的含量（如图附 1－1）。再以此计算供试品中待测元素的含量。

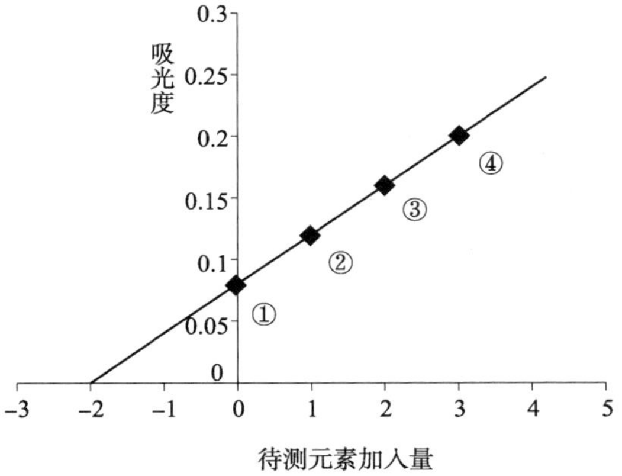

图附 1－1　标准加入法测定待测元素含量示意图

2. 杂质检查法　取供试品，按各品种项下的规定，制备供试品溶液；另取等量的供试品，加入限度量的待测元素溶液，制备成对照品溶液。照上述标准曲线法自“将仪器按规定启动后”操作，并将对照溶液喷入火焰，调节仪器使具合适的读数（a）；在相同的操作条件下喷入供试品溶液，读数（b）；b 值应小于（a－b）。

五、薄层色谱法

薄层色谱法，系将适宜的吸附剂或载体涂布于玻璃板、塑料或铝基片上，成一均匀薄层。待点样、展开后，与适宜的对照物按同法在同板上所得的色谱图对比，并可用薄层扫描仪进行扫描，用以进行药品的鉴别、杂质检查或含量测定的方法。

1. 仪器与材料

（1）玻板　除另有规定外，用 10cm×10cm、10cm×15cm、20cm×10cm 或 20cm×20cm 的规格，要求光滑、平整，洗净后不附水珠，晾干。

（2）吸附剂或载体　最常用的有硅胶 G、硅胶 GF_{254}、硅胶 H、硅胶 HF_{254}、其次有硅藻土、硅藻土 G、氧化铝、氧化铝 G、微晶纤维素、微晶纤维素 F_{254} 等。其颗粒大小一般要求直径为 10～40μm。薄层涂布，除另有规定外，一般可分无黏合剂和含黏合剂两种；前者系将吸附剂或载体用水适量调成糊状，均匀涂布于玻璃板上，后者系在吸附剂或载体中加入一定量的黏合剂，一般常用 10%～15% 的煅石膏（$CaSO_4 \cdot 2H_2O$ 在 140℃加热 4 小时），混匀后加水适量使用，或用羧甲基纤维素钠水溶液（0.2%～0.5%）适量调成糊状，均匀涂布于玻璃板上。也有含一定改性剂如荧光剂或缓冲液等的薄层。

（3）涂布器　应能使吸附剂或载体在玻璃板上手工或自动涂成一层符合厚度要求的均匀薄层。

（4）点样器　一般采用微升毛细管或与之相应的点样器材。

（5）展开室　可用适合薄层板大小的专用玻璃缸，底部平底或有双槽，盖子须密闭。

2. 操作方法

（1）薄层板制备　除另有规定外，将吸附剂 1 份和水 3 份在研钵中向一方向研磨混合，去除表面的气泡后，倒入涂布器中，在玻板上平稳地移动涂布器进行涂布（厚度为 0.25 ~ 0.5mm），取下涂好薄层的玻板，于室温下，置水平台上晾干，在反射光及透射光下检视，表面应均匀，平整，无麻点、无气泡、无破损及污染，于 110℃ 烘 30 分钟，冷却后立即使用或置干燥箱中备用，或用商品预制板。

（2）点样　除另有规定外，用点样器点样于薄层板上，一般为圆点。点样基线距底边 1.0 ~ 1.5cm，样点直径一般不大于 2mm，点间距离可视斑点扩散情况以不影响检出为宜。点样时必须注意勿损伤薄层表面。

（3）展开　将点好样品的薄层板放入展开缸的展开剂中，浸入展开剂的深度为距原点 5mm 为宜，密闭，待展开至规定距离，除另有规定外，一般为 8 ~ 15cm，取出薄层板，晾干，按正文项下的规定检测。

展开缸如需预先用展开剂预平衡，可在缸中加入适量的展开剂，必要时并在壁上贴二条与缸一样高、宽的滤纸条，一端浸入展开剂中，盖严，使展开缸平衡或按正文规定操作。

如需用薄层扫描仪对色谱进行扫描供鉴别、检查或含量测定，则可用薄层扫描法。

3. 薄层扫描法　系指用一定波长的光照射在薄层板上，对薄层色谱中有吸收紫外光或可见光的斑点，或经激发后能发射出荧光的斑点进行扫描，将扫描得到的图谱及积分数据用于药品的鉴别、杂质检查或含量测定。

除另有规定外，薄层扫描方法可根据各种薄层扫描仪的结构特点及使用说明，结合具体情况，选择反射方式，采用吸收法，或荧光法，用双波长或单波长扫描。测定方法有内标法及外标法。由于影响薄层扫描结果的因素很多，故薄层扫描定量测定应在保证供试品斑点的量在校正曲线的线性范围内的情况下，与对照品同板点样，展开，扫描，积分和计算。

用外标法测定时，若对照品各数据点在校正曲线上呈一通过原点的直线时，可用一点法校正，如不通过原点宜采用二点法校正，必要时用多点法校正。含量测定时，供试品溶液和对照品溶液应交叉点于同一薄层板上，供试品点样不得少于 4 个，对照品每一浓度不得少于 2 个，薄层扫描定量用的对照品纯度应符合含量测定用对照品的要求。

六、高效液相色谱法

高效液相色谱法是用高压输液泵将具有不同极性的单一溶剂或不同比例的混合溶剂、缓冲液等流动相泵入装有固定相的色谱柱，经进样阀注入供试品，由流动相带入柱内，在柱内各成分被分离后，依次进入检测器，色谱信号由记录仪或积分仪记录。

1. 对仪器的一般要求　所用的仪器为高效液相色谱仪。色谱柱的填充剂和流动相的组分应按各品种项下的规定。常用的色谱柱填充剂有硅胶和化学键合硅胶，后者以十八烷基硅烷键合硅胶最为常用，辛基硅烷键合硅胶次之，氰基或氨基键合硅胶也有使用。离子交换填充剂，用于离子交换色谱；凝胶或玻璃微球等填充剂，用于分子排阻色谱等。除另有规定外，柱温为室温，检测器为紫外吸收检测器。

在用紫外吸收检测器时。所用流动相应符合紫外分光光度法项下对溶剂的要求。

正文中各品种项下规定的条件除固定相种类、流动相组分、检测器类型不得任意改变外，其余如色谱柱内径、长度、固定相牌号、载体粒度、流动相流速、混合流动相各组分的比例、柱温、进样量、检测器的灵敏度等，均可适当改变，以适应具体品种并达到系统适用性实验的要求。一般色谱图约于20分钟内记录完毕。

2. 系统适用性实验 按各品种项下要求对仪器进行适用性实验，即用规定的对照品对仪器进行试验和调整，应达到规定的要求；或规定分析状态下色谱柱的最小理论板数、分离度、重复性和拖尾因子。

（1）色谱柱的理论板数（n） 在选定的条件下，注入供试品溶液或各品种项下规定的内标物质溶液，记录色谱图，量出供试品主成分或内标物质峰的保留时间 t_R（以分钟或长度计，下同，但应取相同单位）和半峰高（$W_{h/2}$）宽，按 $n = 5.54\ (t_R/W_{h/2})^2$ 计算色谱柱的理论板数。如果测得理论板数低于各品种项下规定的最小理论板数，应改变色谱柱的某些条件（如柱长、载体性能、色谱柱充填的优劣等），使理论板数达到要求。

（2）分离度 定量分析时，为便于准确测量，要求定量峰与其他峰或内标峰之间有较好的分离度。分离度（R）的计算公式为：

$$R = \frac{2(t_{R2} - t_{R1})}{W_1 + W_2}$$

式中 t_{R2}为相邻两峰中后一峰的保留时间；

t_{R1}为相邻两峰中前一峰的保留时间；

W_1及 W_2为此相邻两峰的峰宽。

除另有规定外，分离度应大于1.5。

（3）重复性 取各品种项下的对照溶液，连续进样5次，除另有规定外，其峰面积测量值的相对标准偏差应不大于2.0%。也可按各品种校正因子测定项下，配置相当于80%、100%和120%的对照品溶液，加入规定量的内标溶液，配成3种不同浓度的溶液，分别进样3次，计算平均校正因子，其相对标准偏差也应不大于2.0%。

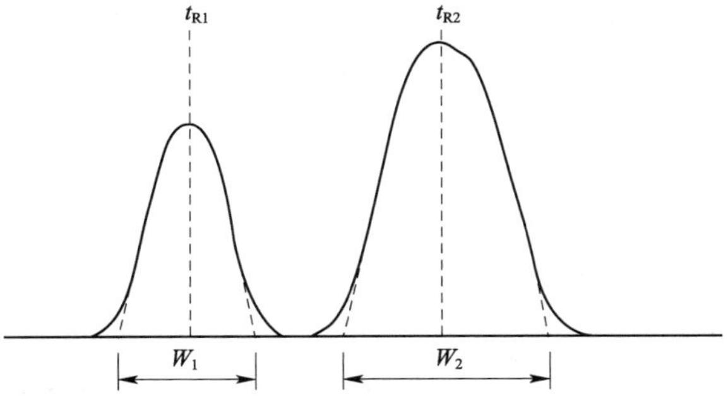

图附1－2 相邻色谱峰分离度的计算

（4）拖尾因子 为保证测量精度，特别当采用峰高法测量时，应检查待测峰的拖尾因子（T）是否符合各品种项下的规定，或不同浓度进样的校正因子误差是否符合要求。拖尾因子计算公式为：

$$T = \frac{W_{0.05h}}{2d_1}$$

式中　$W_{0.05h}$为 0.05 峰高处的峰宽；

d_1为峰极大至峰前沿之间的距离。

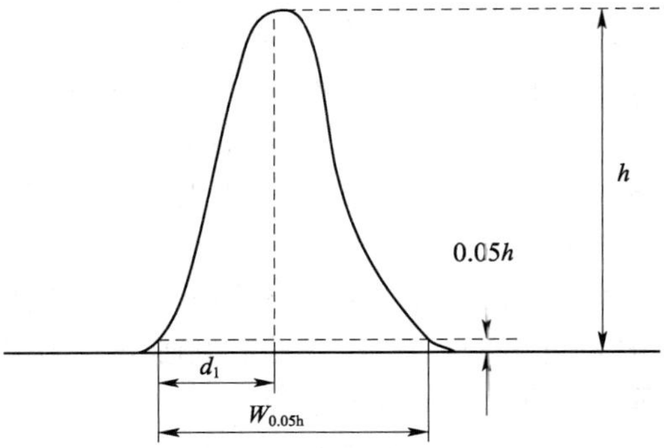

图附 1 - 3　拖尾因子计算方法示意图

除另有规定外，T 应在 0.95 ~ 1.05 之间。

3. 测定法　定量测定时，可根据供试品的具体情况采用峰面积法或峰高法。测定杂质含量时，须采用峰面积法。

（1）内标法加校正因子测定供试品中某个杂质或主成分含量　按各品种项下的规定，精密称（量）取对照品和内标物质，分别配成溶液，精密量取各溶液，配成校正因子测定用的对照溶液。取一定量注入仪器，记录色谱图。测量对照品和内标物质的峰面积或峰高，按下计算校正因子：

$$校正因子（f） = \frac{A_s/C_s}{A_R/C_R}$$

式中　A_s为内标物质的峰面积或峰高；

A_R为对照品的峰面积或峰高；

C_s 为内标物质的浓度；

C_R为对照品的浓度。

再取各品种项下含有内标物质的供试品溶液，注入仪器，记录色谱图，测量供试品中待测成分（或其杂质）和内标物质的峰面积或峰高，按下式计算含量：

$$含量（C_x） = f \cdot \frac{A_x}{A_s/C_s}$$

式中　A_x为供试品（或其杂质）峰面积或峰高；

C_x为供试品（或其杂质）的浓度。

f、A_s和 C_s的意义同上。

当配制校正因子测定用的对照溶液和含有内标物质的供试品溶液使用同一份内标物质溶液时，则配制内标物质溶液不必精密称（量）取。

（2）外标法测定供试品中某个杂质或主成分含量　按各品种项下的规定，精密称（量）取对照品和供试品，配制成溶液，分别精密取一定量，注入仪器，记录色谱图，测量对照品和供试品待测成分的峰面积（或峰高），按下式计算含量：

$$含量（Cx）= C_R \frac{A_x}{A_R}$$

式中各符号意义同上。

（3）加校正因子的主成分自身对照法　测定杂质含量时，可采用加校正因子的主成分自身对照法。在建立方法时，按各品种项下的规定，精密称（量）取杂质对照品和待测成分对照品各适量，配制测定杂质校正因子的溶液，进样，记录色谱图，按上述（1）法计算杂质的校正因子。此校正因子可用于校正杂质的实测峰面积。

测定杂质含量时，按各品种项下规定的杂质限度，将供试品溶液稀释成与杂质限度相当的溶液作为对照溶液，进样，调节仪器灵敏度（以噪音水平可接受为限）或进样量（以柱子不过载为限），使对照溶液的主成分色谱峰高约达满量程的10%～25%或其峰面积能准确积分（面积约为通常条件下满量程峰积分值的10%）。然后，取供试品溶液和对照品溶液适量，分别进样，供试品溶液的记录时间除另有规定外，应为主成分保留时间的若干倍，测量供试品溶液色谱图上各杂质的峰面积，分别乘以相应的校正因子后与对照溶液主成分的峰面积比较，依法计算各杂质含量。

（4）不加校正因子的主成分自身对照法　当没有杂质对照品时，可采用不加校正因子的主成分自身对照法。同上述（3）法配制对照溶液并调节仪器灵敏度后，取供试品溶液和对照溶液适量，分别进样，前者的记录时间除另有规定外，应为主成分保留时间的若干倍，测量供试品溶液色谱图上各杂质的峰面积并与对照溶液主成分的峰面积比较，计算杂质含量。

若供试品所含的部分杂质未与溶剂峰完全分离，则按规定先记录供试品溶液的色谱图Ⅰ，再记录等体积纯溶剂的色谱图Ⅱ。色谱图Ⅰ上杂质峰的总面积（包括溶剂峰），减去色谱图Ⅱ上的溶剂峰面积，即为总杂质峰的校正面积。然后依法计算。

（5）面积归一化法　由于峰面积归一化法测定误差大，因此，本法通常只能用于粗略考察供试品中的杂质含量。除另有规定外，一般不宜用于微量杂质的检查。方法是测量各杂质峰的面积和色谱图上除溶剂峰以外的总色谱峰面积，计算各峰面积占总峰面积的百分率，即得。

由于微量注射器不易精确控制进样量，当采用外标法测定供试品中某杂质或主成分含量时，以定量环进样为好。

（6）一测多评法　中药中所含的有效成分种类复杂，虽然如此，由于生源上的关系，在给定的方法下，他们内在存在着一定的数学关系。利用这些有效成分之间存在的特定函数关系或比例关系，通过测定某一个活性成分，通常该成分为某一中药的化学成分对照品或易于得到的对照品，实现测定一个成分，而达到多个成分通常为对照品难以得到或难供应的，或对照品制备成本高或不稳定的情况下同类多成分同时测定同步测定，这种测定方法为一测多评法。

七、气相色谱法

气相色谱法的流动相为气体，称为载气；色谱柱分为填充柱和毛细管柱两种，填充柱内装吸附剂、高分子多孔小球或涂渍固定液的载体。毛细管柱内壁或载体经涂渍或交联固定液。注入进样口的供试品被加热气化，并被载气带入色谱柱，在柱内各成分被分离后，先后进入检测器，色谱信号用记录仪或数据处理器记录。

1. 对仪器的一般要求 所用的仪器为气相色谱仪。除另有规定外，载气为氮气；色谱柱为填充柱或毛细管柱，填充柱的材质为不锈钢或玻璃，载体用直径为0.25～0.18mm、0.18～0.15mm或0.15～0.125mm经酸洗并硅烷化处理的硅藻土或高分子多孔小球；常用玻璃或弹性石英毛细管柱的内径为0.20mm或0.32mm。进样口温度应高于柱温30～50℃；进样量一般不超过数微升；柱径越细进样量应越少。检测器为氢火焰离子化检测器，检测温度一般高于柱温，并不得低于100℃，以免水汽凝结，通常为250～350℃。

正文中各品种项下规定的条件，除检测器种类、固定液品种及特殊指定的色谱柱材料不得任意改变外，其余如色谱柱内径、长度、载体牌号、粒度、固定液涂布浓度、载气流速、柱温、进样量、检测器的灵敏度等，均可适当改变，以适应具体品种并符合系统适用性试验的要求。一般色谱图约于30分钟内记录完毕。

2. 系统适用性试验 同高效液相色谱法项下规定。

3. 测定法 同高效液相色谱法项下规定。气相色谱法手工进样量不易精确控制，特别应注意留针时间和室温的影响。

附录二 玻璃仪器的洗涤及各种洗液的配制方法

实验中所使用的玻璃仪器清洁与否，直接影响实验结果，往往由于仪器的不清洁或被污染而造成较大的实验误差，甚至会出现相反的实验结果。因此，玻璃仪器的洗涤清洁工作是非常重要的。

1. 初用玻璃仪器的清洗 新购买的玻璃仪器表面常附着有游离的碱性物质，可先用肥皂水（或去污粉）洗刷再用自来水洗净，然后浸泡在1%～2%盐酸溶液中过夜（不少于4小时），再用自来水冲洗，最后用蒸馏水冲洗2～3次，在100～130°C烘箱中烤干备用。

2. 用过的玻璃仪器的清洗

（1）一般玻璃仪器 如试管、烧杯、锥形瓶等（包括量筒），先用自来水洗刷至无污物，再选用大小合适的毛刷沾取去污粉（掺入肥皂粉）或浸入肥皂水内。将器皿内外（特别是内壁）细心刷洗，用自来水冲洗干净后，蒸馏水冲洗2～3次，烤干或倒置在清洁处，干后备用。凡洗净的玻璃器皿，不应在器壁上带有水珠，否则表示尚未洗干净，应再按上述方法重新洗涤。若发现内壁有难以去掉的污迹，应分别试用下述各种洗涤剂予以清除，再重新冲洗。

（2）量器 如吸量管、滴定管、量瓶等。使用后应立即浸泡于凉水中，勿使物质干涸。工作完毕后用流水冲洗，以除去附着的试剂、蛋白质等物质，晾干后浸泡在铬酸溶液中4～6小时（或过夜），再用自来水充分冲洗，最后用蒸馏水冲洗2～4次，风干备用。

（3）其他 具有传染性样品的容器，如病毒、传染病患者的血清等沾污过的容器，应先进行高压（或其他方法）消毒后再进行清洗，盛过各种有毒试剂，特别是剧毒药品和放射性同位素物质的容器，必须经过专门处理（略），确知没有残余毒物存在方可进行清洗。

3. 洗涤液的种类和配制方法

（1）铬酸洗液（重铬酸钾－硫酸洗液，或简称为洗液） 广泛用于玻璃仪器的洗涤，常用的配制方法有下述四种：

①取 100ml 工业浓硫酸置于烧杯内，小心加热，然后小心慢慢加入 5g 重铬酸钾粉末，边加边搅拌，待全部溶解后冷却，贮于具玻璃塞的细口瓶内。

②称取 5g 重铬酸钾粉末置于 250ml 烧杯中，加水 5ml，尽量使其溶解，慢慢加入浓硫酸 100ml，随加随搅拌，冷却后贮存备用。

③称取 80 克重铬酸钾，溶于 1000ml 自来水中，慢慢加入工业硫酸 100ml（边加边用玻璃棒搅拌）。

④称取 200 克重铬酸钾，溶于 500ml 自来水中，慢慢加入工业硫酸 500ml（边加边搅拌）。

（2）浓盐酸（工业用） 可洗去水垢或某些无机盐沉淀。

（3）5%草酸溶液 用数滴硫酸酸化，可洗去高锰酸钾的痕迹。

（4）5%～10%磷酸三钠（$Na_3PO_4 \cdot 12H_2O$）溶液 可洗去油污物。

（5）30%硝酸溶液 洗涤 CO_2测定仪器及微量滴管。

（6）5%～10%乙二胺四乙酸二钠（$EDTA-Na_2$）溶液 加热煮沸可洗玻璃仪器内壁的白色沉淀物。

（7）尿素洗涤液 为蛋白质的良好溶剂，适用于洗涤盛蛋白质制剂及血样的容器。

（8）酒精与浓硝酸混合液 最适合于洗净滴定管，在滴定管中加入 3ml 酒精，然后沿管口慢慢加入 4ml 浓硝酸（比重 1.4），盖住滴定管管口，利用所产生的氧化氮洗净滴定管。

（9）有机溶剂 如丙酮、乙醇、乙醚等可用于洗脱油脂、脂溶性染料等污痕。二甲苯可洗脱油漆的污垢。

（10）氢氧化钾的乙醇溶液和含有高锰酸钾的氢氧化钠溶液 是两种强碱性的洗涤液，对玻璃仪器的侵蚀性很强，清除容器内壁污垢，洗涤时间不宜过长，使用时应小心慎重。

上述洗涤液可多次使用，使用前必须将待洗涤之玻璃仪器先用水冲洗多次，除去肥皂去污粉或各种废液。若仪器上有凡士林或羊毛脂时，应先用软纸擦去，然后用乙醇或乙醚擦净后才能使用洗液，否则会使洗涤液迅速失效。例如：肥皂水，有机溶液（乙醇、甲醛等）及少量油污皆会使重铬酸钾－硫酸洗液变绿，减低洗涤能力。

附录三 常用溶剂性质

表中列出了最重要的有机溶剂，在数值上按 ε^{o}增加次序排列，在测定 ε^{o}时，Snyder 以正戊烷为参比溶剂（$\varepsilon^{o}=0.00$），然后测定标准品在不同溶剂作为流动相时的保留体积。从本质上看，此系列中溶剂的次序按照组分在固定相上吸附能力减小的次序排列，即使用第一种溶剂时，组分的 K 值最大，而使用最后一种溶剂时，由于它的洗脱能力极高，以致组分不被滞留。

表附 3-1 常用溶剂的性质

溶剂名称	沸点（℃）	ε^{o}（硅胶）	电解常数	黏度 η（20℃）	折光率（R_2）	UV 截止波长（nm）	溶解度（20~25℃）	
							溶剂在水中（%）	水在溶剂中（%）
正戊烷	33	0.00		0.23	1.358	205		
正己烷	69	0.00	1.88	0.33	1.375	195	0.00095	0.0111
异辛烷		+0.01		0.50	1.404	197		
环己烷	81	0.03	2.02	1.00	1.427	205	0.010	0.0055
戊烯-1		+0.06		0.18	1.371	-		
二硫化碳	46	+0.11	2.64	0.37	1.626	380	0.294	<0.005
四氯化碳	77	+0.14	2.24	0.97	1.466	265	0.077	0.010
二甲苯	137	+0.20	2.38	0.6~0.8	-1.5	290	0.0176	0.5402
异丙醚	68	+0.22		0.37	1.368	220		
氯异丙烷	47	+0.22		0.33	1.378	225		
甲苯	110	+0.22	2.37	0.59	1.496	285	0.1515	0.0334
苯	80	+0.25	2.29	0.65	1.501	280	0.1780	0.063
乙醚	35	+0.29	4.34	0.23	1.353	220	0.042	1.468
三氯甲烷	61	+0.31	4.81	0.57	1.443	245	0.815	0.072
二氯甲烷	40	+0.32		0.44	1.424	233		
四氢呋喃	66	+0.35	7.58	—	1.408	220	任意	混溶
二氯乙烯		+0.38		0.79	1.445	230		
丙酮	56	+0.43	2.07	+0.32	1.359	330	溶解	度大
二氧六环	101	+0.43	2.21	1.54	1.422	220	任意	混溶
乙酸乙酯	77	+0.45	6.02	0.45	1.370	260	8.0	2.94
戊醇	138		13.9	4.1	1.410	210	2.19	7.41
二甲亚砜	189	+0.48		2.24	1.479	-		
乙腈	82	+0.50	37.5	0.37	1.344	190	任意	混溶
吡啶	115	+0.55	12.3	0.94	1.510	305		
异丙醇	82	+0.63	19.92	2.3	1.38	205	任意	混溶
正丙醇	97	+0.63	20.3	2.3	1.38	205	任意	混溶
乙醇	78	+0.68	24.3	1.20	1.361	210	任意	混溶
甲醇	64	0.73	33.6	0.60	1.329	205	任意	混溶
乙酸	118	大	6.15	1.26	1.37	-	任意	混溶
水	100	大	80.4	1.00	1.333	195	任意	混溶

附录四　色谱法预试中药化学成分

色谱法常用来进一步确证定性实验呈正反应的各类化学成分。它是将上述正结果的供试液进行适当的浓缩，再按可能含有的某类化学成分的一般色谱条件进行薄层色谱或纸上色谱分离，最后进行该类化合物的显色反应，观察结果，这样可以排除一部分其他化合物的干扰，各类成分的色谱条件参阅下表。

表附4-1　各类成分色谱预试条件

化合物	色谱条件		检测方法		附注
	吸附剂或载体	展开剂	显色剂	结果	
生物碱	氧化铝-CMC	苯，三氯甲烷，乙酸乙酯，乙醇等单一溶剂；氯仿-甲醇（9:1）；苯-乙醇（8:2）	改良碘化铋钾	橙红色斑点	碱性生物碱在选用纸色谱或薄层色谱时，可选用碱性展开剂或将硅胶板氨气饱和后展开。碱性弱的生物碱可选用吸附薄层色谱
	硅胶-CMC	氯仿-二乙胺（NH_4OH）(9:1)；三氯甲烷-丙酮-二乙胺（5:4:1）			
	层析滤纸	正丁醇-醋酸-水（4:1:5）（上层）；乙酸乙酯：吡啶：水（2:1:2）	观察荧光	各种荧光斑点	
糖和多糖	层析滤纸	正丁醇-醋酸-水（4:1:5）（上层）；乙酸乙酯-吡啶-水（2:1:2）	茴香醛 氨性硝酸银	不同颜色的斑点；棕黑色斑点	氨性硝酸银需加热至110℃方能显色 主要用于检出还原糖
酚类鞣质	层析滤纸 硅胶-CMC	正丁醇-醋酸-水（4:1:5）（上层）；三氯甲烷-丙酮（9:1）	三氯化铁 三氯化铁-铁氰化钾（1:1）	蓝、绿、黑等各色斑点	
黄酮	硅胶-CMC	三氯甲烷-甲醇-丙酮（40:25:35）；乙酸乙酯-丁醇-丙酮-水（3:3:1:1）	10% Na_2CO_3水液、氨气熏、10% $AlCl_3$醇液（喷试剂前后观察荧光）	观察喷洒Na_2CO_3氨熏前后荧光的变化，多为黄色或黄绿色荧光斑点	在醋酸水系统中可区分苷或苷元，苷元多在原点，苷可展开；在正丁醇-醋酸-水系统中苷元的R_f值较苷大
	层析滤纸	15%醋酸水-正丁醇-醋酸-水（4:1:5）（上层）			
	聚酰胺	甲醇-水（8:2）；乙醇-水（3:2）；丙酮-水（1:1）			

续表

化合物	色谱条件		检测方法		附注
	吸附剂或载体	展开剂	显色剂	结果	
蒽醌	硅胶-CMC	苯-乙酸乙酯（3∶17）；乙酸乙酯-甲醇-水（100∶1.65∶1.35）；三氯甲烷-乙醇（75∶25）；石油醚-丙酮-水（5∶3∶1）	1%～2%的苛性碱醇溶液 0.5% $MgAC_2$ 甲醇液（90℃加热5分钟）	红色斑点、橙红、紫红色斑点	硅胶色谱条件适应于游离蒽醌的检出纸色谱对苷也可以展开
香豆素萜类内酯	硅胶-CMC	甲苯-乙酸乙酯-甲酸（5∶4∶1）；石油醚-乙酸乙酯（5∶1）；正丁醇-醋酸-水（4∶1∶5）	观察荧光	蓝绿色荧光	香豆素类苷可在硅胶板上为正丁醇-醋酸-水（4∶1∶5）所展开
	酸性氧化铝	石油醚-三氯甲烷（1∶1）；石油醚-乙醚（1∶1）	重氮化试剂	红紫色斑点	
	层析滤纸	正丁醇-醋酸-水（4∶1∶5）	观察荧光	蓝绿色荧光	
强心苷	滑石粉-石膏（7∶3）（甲酰胺为固定相）	三氯甲烷-丙酮-乙酸乙酯（8∶2∶0.5∶2.5），甲酰胺饱和	碱性3，5-二硝基苯甲酸	红色、紫色斑点（110℃烘5分钟）	此处列出的条件中滑石粉板适合于含糖分子较多的强心苷分离。对于苷元或糖分子较少的强心苷的分离可用另两种条件，或一般的吸附色谱条件（同甾体）
	硅胶-CMC	二氯甲烷-甲醇-甲酰胺（80∶19∶1）；氯仿-甲醇-乙酸（85∶13∶2）；乙酸乙酯-吡啶-水（5∶1∶4）	氯胺T-三氯乙酸试剂	浅蓝色背景呈橙红色斑点（烘5分钟）	
	层析滤纸（甲酰胺为固定相）	苯；甲苯-三氯甲烷-甲酰胺（6∶4 饱和）	碱性苦味酸试剂	橙红色斑点（110℃烘5分钟）	

附录五　常用色谱显色剂及使用

一、通用显色剂

1. 碘蒸气　将薄层板放入底部有少许结晶碘片的密闭容器（可在广口瓶内于水浴上进行），碘则迅速升华，碘蒸气充满整个空间，能使许多化合物在淡黄的背景上产生棕色斑点。

2. 硫酸

（1）50%硫酸的甲醇溶液（将等体积的浓硫酸与甲醇于冷却的条件下小心混合）。

（2）5%浓硫酸的乙醇溶液。

（3）15%浓硫酸的正丁醇溶液。

（4）5%浓硫酸的醋酐溶液。

（5）50%浓硫酸的醋酸溶液。

薄层板用上述试剂之一喷雾，在空气中干燥15分钟，然后于110℃加热直到展现的颜色或荧光达到最大强度为止。对于含CMC－Na黏合剂的薄层板不宜用此类检定剂，因加热时可使背景发黑而干扰观察。

注：胆甾醇、维生素A及其酯以及许多异戊间二烯类脂化合物，用（1）项下试剂喷雾后加热，易出现特殊颜色，胆甾醇和其酯类由红色、红紫色最后转变为棕色，维生素A和其酯类最初呈蓝色，许多化合物接着碳化，产生黑色斑点。

3. 碱性高锰酸钾 1%高锰酸钾溶液与0.5%碳酸钠溶液等体积混合，喷雾，还原性物质在淡红色背景下显蓝色。

4. 碘溶液 0.5%碘的三氯甲烷溶液，对很多化合物显黄棕色。

5. 碘－碘化钾 0.2g碘、0.4g碘化钾溶于100ml水中，许多化合物可以与其显黄棕色。

6. 磷钼酸试剂 5%磷钼酸的醇溶液，喷后于120℃烘烤，还原性物质显蓝色，再用氨气熏，则背景变成红色。

7. 磷钨酸试剂 20%磷钨酸的乙醇溶液，喷后于120℃烘烤，还原性物质显蓝色。

8. 铁氰化钾－三氯化铁 1%铁氰化钾与2%三氯化铁等量混合喷雾，还原性物质显蓝色，若再喷2M 2N盐酸溶液，则颜色加深。

9. 荧光检定剂

（1）0.2% 2′，7－二氯荧光素乙醇溶液。

（2）0.01%荧光素乙醇溶液。

（3）0.1%桑色素乙醇溶液。

（4）0.05% 罗丹明B乙醇溶液。

喷以上任一溶液，不同的物质可能在荧光背景上显黑色或其他颜色斑点。

（5）荧光素（钠）溶液：50mg荧光素钠（又称荧光黄钠）溶于100ml 50%甲醇中，喷后于紫外光下观察，为芳香和杂环化合物的通用检定剂。

二、生物碱及含氮化合物

1. 碘化铋钾试剂

（1）溶液Ⅰ 0.85g次硝酸铋溶于10ml冰醋酸与40ml水中。

（2）溶液Ⅱ 8g碘化钾溶于20ml水中。

（3）贮备液 溶液Ⅰ与溶液Ⅱ等体积混合，可于棕色瓶中保存较长时间，一般贮备液可作沉淀剂用。

（4）喷雾剂 1ml贮备液与2ml乙酸、10ml水混合而得。生物碱可与之显橘红色斑点。

2. 改良碘化铋钾－Ⅰ

（1）贮备液 将8g碱式硝酸铋溶于20～23ml 25%硝酸中，将此液边搅拌边缓慢地加入到由20g碘化钾1ml 6M盐酸和5ml水组成的混悬液中，再加水至深色沉淀中，直到变成橘红色溶液为止。本溶液体积约为95ml，滤去不溶性残渣后，加水稀释至100ml，贮备于深色容器中，于冰箱中可保存数周。

（2）喷雾剂　下列溶液依次混合即可。20ml水，6ml 6M盐酸，2ml贮备液，6ml 6M氢氧化钠液。若氢氧化铋振摇后不溶解，可加数滴6M盐酸。该喷雾剂于冰箱中可保存10日左右，用于含季铵氮的化合物。

3. 碘化汞钾试剂　13.55g氯化汞和49.8g碘化钾各溶于20ml水中，混合后稀释至1000ml，再加入1/10体积的17%盐酸即可用于喷雾。

注：该试剂可用作生物碱沉淀剂。

4. 酸性碘－碘化钾　将1g碘和10g碘化钾于5ml水中加热溶解，再加2ml醋酸，用水稀释至100ml即可。

5. 铁氰化钾－亚铁氰化钾　将57mg铁氰化钾和7.8mg亚铁氰化钾溶于100ml蒸馏水中即可，用于检定吗啡。

6. 高氯酸－氯化铁　将100ml 5%高氯酸水溶液、2ml 0.05M氢氧化铁溶液混合即可用于喷雾。检定吲哚衍生物，但靛红和2－羟基吲哚衍生物不发生反应。

7. 硅钨酸试剂　将1g硅钨酸溶于20ml水中，加10%盐酸使呈酸性即得，用作生物碱的沉淀剂。

8. 磷钨酸试剂

（1）喷雾剂　为5%～10%磷钨酸的乙醇溶液，喷后于120℃加热。

（2）沉淀剂　磷钼酸钠20g溶于硝酸中，加水使成10%。

9. 对－二甲氨基苯甲醛－硫酸

（1）将125mg对－二甲氨基苯甲醛溶于65ml硫酸和35ml水的混合液中，放冷，加入0.05ml 5%三氯化铁水溶液，此试液，可保存一周，用于检测麦角生物碱。

（2）0.5%对－二甲氨基苯甲醛乙醇溶液与浓硫酸以5∶1混合即可，喷后有时需于80℃加热几分钟，生物碱显红或橙色斑，麦角生物碱显蓝色斑。

（3）0.5%对－二甲氨基苯甲醛的环己烷溶液，喷后生物碱显红或橙色斑点，麦角生物碱显蓝色斑点。

三、糖类

1. 苯胺－邻苯二甲酸　将0.93g苯胺和1.66g邻苯二甲酸溶解在100ml水饱和的正丁醇中即得。喷雾后于105℃加热10分钟。不同种类的糖会出现不同颜色的斑点，戊醛糖显红色，己醛、甲基戊糖醛、糖醛酸显褐色，己酮糖显淡褐色，在紫外灯光下观察荧光更清楚，该试剂受杂质干扰影响较小，对还原糖的检出灵敏度高。

2. 对－茴香胺－邻苯二甲酸　为0.1M对茴香胺和邻苯二甲酸的95%乙醇溶液。喷雾后于100℃加热10分钟，己糖显绿色，6－去氧己糖显黄绿色，戊糖显红紫色，糖醛酸显棕色。

3. 苯胺－磷酸　将2M以水饱和的苯胺正丁醇溶液，加1M磷酸正丁醇溶液（1∶2，v/v）即得。喷雾后于105℃加热10分钟。

4. 苯胺－二苯胺－磷酸　将4g二苯胺、4ml苯胺和20ml 85%磷酸溶解于200ml

丙酮中即可，喷雾后于85℃加热10分钟，此试剂对还原糖产生各种颜色，1，4–己醛糖、低聚糖变成蓝色。

5. 联苯胺试剂 将0.5g联苯胺溶于20ml冰醋酸和80ml无水醇中，喷到纸上于110℃左右加热，糖出现褐色斑点。

6. 1，3–二羟基萘酚–磷酸 0.2%1，3–二羟基萘酚乙醇溶液100ml与85%磷酸100ml混匀后使用，喷后105℃烤5～10分钟，酮糖显红色，醛糖显淡蓝色。

7. 3，5二氨基苯甲酸–磷酸 取3，5–二氨基苯甲酸溶于80%磷酸中，并用60ml水稀释之即可，层析板喷雾后于100℃加热15分钟，在长波紫外光下，斑点显黄色～绿荧光，日光下呈棕色，可检出2μg以上的量，用于检测α–脱氧糖。

8. 萘骈间苯二酚–硫酸

（1）溶液Ⅰ 0.2%萘骈间苯二酚的乙醇溶液。

（2）溶液Ⅱ 20%硫酸。

使用前，将Ⅰ与Ⅱ等体积混合之，喷后100～105℃加热5～10分钟，用于糖类检测。

9. α–萘酚–硫酸 为10.5ml 15% α–萘酚溶液、65ml浓硫酸、40.5ml乙醇以及4ml水的混合溶液。喷后于100℃加热3～6分钟。

10. 茴香醛–硫酸试剂 浓硫酸1ml加到含茴香醛0.5ml的50ml乙醇溶液中（临用前鲜配）即可，喷后100～105℃加热，各种糖显不同颜色。

11. 蒽酮 将0.38g蒽酮溶解于10ml醛酸和20ml乙醇中，再加3ml 85%磷酸和1ml水即可（此溶液在冰箱中可保存数周）。喷后110℃加热5～6分钟后，酮糖和含酮糖的低聚糖出现黄色斑点。

12. 尿酸–盐酸 5g尿素溶于20ml 2N盐酸中，再加100ml乙醇即得，喷后薄层板于100℃加热直至出现最佳颜色。酮糖和含酮糖的低聚糖转为成蓝色。

13. 费林试剂

（1）溶液Ⅰ 硫酸铜溶液，溶解34.66g硫酸铜于水中，并稀释至500ml。

（2）溶液Ⅱ 碱性酒石酸盐溶液，溶解173g酒石酸钾和50g氢氧化钠于水中，再稀释至冷时为500ml，临用时，两液等体积混合。用于检测还原糖。

14. 醋酸酮试剂 溶解66g醋酸铜和10ml冰醋酸于水中，稀释至1L即可。用于检测还原单糖。

四、酚类化合物

1. 重氮化试剂

（1）重氮盐的制备 取50g对氨基苯磺酸溶于250ml 10%的氢氧化钠溶液中，一面冷却一面滴加10%的亚硝钠溶液200ml。另外在80ml浓盐酸中加入40ml水并用冰水冷却后滴加到上述溶液中，即生成重氮盐沉淀，过滤，用冰水、乙醇、乙醚依次洗涤沉淀物，风干即得纯重氮盐。

（2）喷雾剂 取0.1g纯重氮盐溶于20ml 10%氢氧化钠中，即可喷雾，在滤纸上酚类化合物物呈现红色斑点。

2. 重氮化氨基苯磺酸试剂 对氨基本磺酸0.9g，加热溶于9ml 12M盐酸中，用水稀释到100ml，取此溶液10ml用水冷却，加入冰冷的4.5%亚硝酸钠溶液10ml，0℃放15分钟（0℃可保存3天），用前加等体积1%碳酸钠溶液即可，喷后香豆精显黄、橙、红棕、紫等颜色，也用于酚类、芳香胺及能偶合的杂环化合物的检验。

3. 重氮化对硝基苯胺试剂 取对硝基苯胺0.7g溶于12M盐酸9ml，用水稀释到100ml，将此溶液4ml逐滴加入到冰冷的1%亚硝酸钠溶液5ml中，再用冰冷的水稀释至100ml即可（临用时鲜配），喷后香豆精显黄、橙、红、棕、紫等颜色，也用于酚类显色。

4. 重氮化联苯胺

（1）联苯胺贮备液 5g联苯胺和14ml 36%盐酸混合，加水稀释至1000ml。

（2）亚硝酸盐溶液 为10%亚硝酸钠的水溶液，临用前现配。

（3）喷雾剂 在0℃条件下，将20ml联苯胺溶液和20ml亚硝酸钠溶液混合，且不断搅拌（本试剂仅能保存2～3小时），喷后不同酚的颜色可迅速出现或在几小时后才出现。

5. 重氮化磺胺酸 4.5g磺酸溶于45ml温热的12M盐酸中，并用水稀释至500ml，取此稀释液于冰中冷却，加入10ml 4.5%亚硝酸钠冷溶液，本试剂于0℃保持15分钟，本喷雾剂临用前应加等体积10%磺酸钠水溶液，用于检测酚类、胺类及能偶合的杂环化合物。

6. 间苯三酚－浓硫酸试剂 为2%间苯三酚乙醇溶液与浓硫酸的等体积混合液，用于检测原儿茶醛。

7. 三氯化铁试剂 1%～5%三氯化铁的0.5M盐酸的水或乙醇溶液，酚类呈蓝色或绿色，本试剂还可用作试管与点滴反应。

8. 铁氰化钾－氯化铁 将1%铁氰化钾水溶液同2%氯化铁水溶液于使用前等体积混合即可。喷后再喷以2M盐酸，色泽可以增强，用于检测酚类、胺类、硫代硫盐酸和异硫氰酸盐，还可用于阿魏酸的定量测定。

9. 三氯化铝试剂 为1%三氯化铝乙醇液或5%三氯化铝水溶液，用于检测黄酮，试管检识与喷雾均可。

10. 三氯化锑试剂 为10%三氯化锑的三氯甲烷溶液，喷雾后，黄酮可在长波紫外光下产生黄色荧光斑点。

11. 4－氨基匹林铁氰化钾

（1）喷雾剂Ⅰ 为2%4－氨基匹林乙醇溶液。

（1）喷雾剂Ⅱ 为8%铁氰化钾水溶液。

方法：分别用喷雾剂Ⅰ、Ⅱ喷后，将层析谱放入含有25%氢氧化铵的密闭容器中显示红橙～淡红斑点，用于检测酚类、香豆精。

12. 碱性醋酸铅 为避25%碱性醋酸铅的水溶液，喷后在长波紫外光下观察荧光，用于检测黄酮类化合物。

13. 硫酸铜柠檬酸钠 1.73g硫酸铜（$CuSO_4 \cdot 5H_2O$），1.73g柠檬酸钠和10g无水碳酸钠溶于水中，加水至100ml即可，用于检测黄酮、邻二羟基香豆素。

注：有邻二羟基基团的化合物，在长波紫外光下的荧光可被喷雾剂所减弱或完全熄灭，而不具此基团的这类化合物是不改变的，甚至可增强（在此情况下，通常发生荧光颜色的变化）。

五、醌类化合物

1. 醋酸镁试剂　为0.5%醋酸镁的甲醇溶液喷后于90℃加热5分钟即可显色，该反应灵敏，邻位酚羟基蒽醌呈紫～蓝紫色；对位二酚羟基蒽醌呈紫红～紫色；每个苯环上各有一个α－羟基或有间位羟基者，呈橙红～红色；母核只有一个α或一个β－酚羟基者，或者有两个β－酚羟基但不在同环上，呈黄橙色至橙色。

2. 3%氢氧化钠或碳酸钠溶液　以此试剂喷雾或进行试管反应均可。

3. 无色亚甲蓝试剂　将含有0.25g锌粉的1ml醋酸混悬液加入5ml的0.02%的亚甲蓝丙酮溶液中即可，用于检测醌类（一般、结合）和生育醌。

4. 氢氧化钾试剂　为5%氢氧化钾甲醇溶液，层析谱干燥后可在日光和长波紫外光下检识，用于检测香豆精、蒽醌及其苷。

5. 对－亚硝基二甲苯胺试剂　为0.1%对－亚硝基二甲苯胺的吡啶溶液，可与羟基蒽醌类化合物，尤其是9，12未取代的1，8－二羟基蒽酮生成紫红、绿、蓝以及灰、亮红、紫等不同颜色，随分子结构不同而异，不仅可用于蒽酮类化合物定性，而且还可用于微量定量。

6. 哌啶试剂　为50%哌啶的苯溶液。

7. 乙酸铝试剂　为0.5%乙酸铝溶液。

8. 碳酸锂试剂　为饱和的碳酸锂溶液。

9. 硼砂试剂　为饱和的硼砂溶液。

六、萜类化合物

1. 碘蒸气　见一.1，可检测香茶菜、冬凌草中的二萜Oridonin等及烃基马桑毒素等多种有机化合物。

2. 磷钼酸试剂　为10%磷钼酸的乙醇溶液，用于检测马桑毒素（Oriamyrtin）等。

3. 香草醛－硫酸试剂　1%香草醛的浓硫酸溶液或1%香草醛的50%磷酸溶液，喷后加热至显色，于日光和紫外光下观察，用于检测萜烯类。

4. 无水氯化铁试剂　为饱和的无水氯化铁甲醇溶液，用于检定萜烯类。

5. 对－二甲氨基苯甲醛－磷酸　1g对－二甲氨基苯甲醛溶解于5g浓磷酸和50ml冰醋酸中，用水稀释至100ml，贮于棕色瓶中，喷后100℃加热几分钟，薁类显深蓝色斑。

6. 香草醛－高氯酸试剂　5ml 10%香草醛的冰醋酸溶液与1ml高氯酸临用时混合，喷后加热烘烤至显色，用于检测倍半萜莪术醇（Carcumol）等。

七、挥发油

1. 硫酸　13%硫酸喷后110℃加热至显色，不适用于带有CMC－Na的薄层板。

2. 香草醛－硫酸

（1）1%香草醛的浓硫酸溶液。

（2）0.5%香草醛的硫酸－乙醇（4∶1）溶液。

（3）5%香草醛的浓硫酸溶液。

喷后于120℃加热或红外灯烘烤，直到取得最大程度的色斑为止，可出现各种颜色，反应灵敏。

3. 香草醛－盐酸 为5%香草醛的浓盐酸溶液，喷后于120℃加热，挥发油中各成分可呈现各种颜色。

4. 茴香醛－浓硫酸试剂

（1）浓硫酸1ml加入50ml冰乙酸中，加茴香醛0.5ml，必须临用时新配。

（2）茴香醛－浓硫酸－乙醇（1∶1∶18）配成喷雾剂，以上二试剂之一喷雾，喷后于105℃烘烤，可使挥发油中各成分显不同颜色。

5. 荧光素－溴试剂

（1）溶液Ⅰ：0.1%荧光素的乙醇溶液。

（2）溶液Ⅱ：5%溴的四氯化碳溶液。

方法：薄层板喷溶液Ⅰ后，放入盛溶液Ⅱ的槽中，溴将荧光素转变成粉红色的曙红（cosin），它在长波紫外光下不显荧光，如果薄层上有乙烯基化合物，则溴与它作用而不与荧光素作用，在长波紫外光下观察时，此处仍显荧光素的黄色荧光。

6. 异羟肟酸铁试剂

（1）溶液Ⅰ：5%盐酸羟胺溶于12ml水中，再用乙醇稀释到50ml，储于冷处。

（2）溶液Ⅱ：10g氢氧化钠溶于少量水中，再用乙醇稀释到100ml。

（3）溶液Ⅲ：溶液Ⅰ和溶液Ⅱ以1∶2混合，滤出氯化钾沉淀，所得滤液必须放冰箱中，可稳定两周。

（4）溶液Ⅳ：10g三氯化铁溶于20ml 36%盐酸中，与200ml乙醚振摇，得均匀的溶液，密塞储存可长久使用。

用法：先喷溶液Ⅲ，于室温稍干燥后，再喷溶液Ⅳ，喷后斑点显淡红色，可能是挥发油中的酯和内酯。

7. 2，4－二硝基苯肼

（1）0.4%2，4－二硝基苯肼的2M 2N盐酸溶液。

（2）将1g 2，4－二硝基苯肼溶于1000ml乙醇中，加入10ml 36%盐酸即得。

以二试剂之一喷雾，饱和酮类与2，4－二硝基苯肼可立即产生蓝色，饱和醛则作用较慢并转变成草绿色，不饱和羟基化合物的色泽只是慢慢地改变或根本不发生变化，用于特定挥发油中羟基化合物。

8. 邻联二茴香胺试剂 0.3%邻联二茴香胺的冰醋酸溶液，喷后如呈现黄色斑点，表明样品中含有醛。

八、甾体化合物

1. 醋酐－浓硫酸 在冷却条件下，小心地将5ml醋酐同5ml浓硫酸混合，同样在冷却情况下，将此混合物谨慎地加入50ml无水乙醇中，临用前现配，喷后100℃干燥10分钟，置长波紫外光下观察，用于检测甾醇、三萜皂苷及甾醇类。

2. 肉桂醛－醋酐－硫酸

（1）喷雾剂Ⅰ：1%肉桂醛的乙醇溶液。

（2）喷雾剂Ⅱ：醋酐与浓硫酸的12∶1（v/v）混合液，临用前现配。

薄层板以喷雾剂Ⅰ喷后，于90℃干燥5分钟，再喷Ⅱ，于室温放置1～2分钟后，移放于干燥箱中，再于90℃加热至斑点出现为止，用于检测甾体皂苷。

3. 硫酸高铈－硫酸 为硫酸高铈的65%硫酸饱和溶液，喷后于120℃加热15分钟，用于检测茄属甾体生物碱和甾体皂苷。

注：不能用于氧化铝薄层板。

4. 茴香醛－浓硫酸试剂 见七.5。喷后于100～105℃加热，直至色斑呈最大强度为止。粉红色斑暴露于水蒸气中时色泽褪去。地衣成分、酚类、萜类、糖类和甾体化合物可根据分别呈紫、蓝、红、灰和绿色斑来检测。

改良喷雾剂：为新配的0.5%茴香酮、9ml乙醇、0.5ml浓硫酸和0.1ml醋酸混合液，可用于检测含糖物质，喷后于90～100℃加热5～10分钟。

5. 氯磺酸－醋酸 5ml氯磺酸在冷却条件下，溶于10ml醋酸中，喷后于130℃加热5～10分钟，在长波紫外光下可见到荧光，用于检测三萜与甾体化合物。

6. 三氯醋酸

（1）25%三氯醋酸的氯仿溶液。

（2）1%三氯醋酸的氯仿溶液（检查维生素B）。

（3）3.3g三氯醋酸溶于10ml氯仿中，再加1～2滴30%过氧化氢（H_2O_2）即可。

以上三试剂喷雾后，于120℃加热5～10分钟，色斑在日光和长波紫外光下可检出，用于检测甾体、洋地黄毒苷、藜芦生物碱。

7. 三氟乙酸 1%三氟乙酸的氯仿溶液，喷后于120℃加热5分钟，用于检测甾体化合物。

8. 三氯化锑－醋酸 将20g三氯化锑溶解于20ml醋酸和60ml氯仿的混合液中，喷后于100℃加热5分钟，在紫外光下观察，用于检测甾体、二萜类化合物，后者出现红黄～蓝紫的色斑。

9. 五氯化锑 25%五氯化锑的氯仿或四氯化碳溶液，用前鲜配，喷后于120℃加热，直到色斑出现，在长波紫外光下检之，用于检测甾体皂苷、萜类、油脂、树脂、维生素A、D、E。

10. 氯化锌 30%氯化锌的甲醇溶液，溶后过滤即得，喷后将薄层板于105℃加热1小时，然后立即用一玻璃板覆盖，以防止湿气对其影响，色斑在长波紫外光下可见荧光，用于检测甾体和甾体皂苷。

11. 高氯酸 20%高氯酸水溶液。用于甾体。喷后于150℃加热约10分钟，直至形成最显著色斑，在长波紫外光下可观察到荧光。

12. 氢氧化钠 10%氢氧化钠溶液，喷后于80℃干燥10分钟于紫外光下观察，$\triangle^4$－3－酮甾族化合物显黄色荧光。

九、氨基酸

1. 茚三酮试剂

（1）茚三酮0.3g溶于正丁醇100ml中，加冰醋酸3ml。

（2）茚三酮0.2g溶于乙醇100ml中。

用上述试剂之一喷雾，喷后于110℃加热至显出颜色，为了使茚三酮的显色稳定，可采用下法：用茚三酮试剂显色后，用硝酸铜试剂（饱和硝酸铜溶液1ml与10%硝酸溶液0.2ml及96%乙醇100ml混合）喷，斑点由蓝紫色转为红色。

（3）茚三酮浸泡显色法，把配成0.25%的茚三酮丙酮溶液（99%以上的无水丙酮）放在瓷盘内，把展开后的滤纸浸到丙酮溶液中，取出后风干，于90℃加热显色，此法干燥迅速，显色快，颜色均匀鲜艳。

2. 茚三酮－硝酸铜试剂

（1）溶液Ⅰ：将10ml醋酸和2ml可力丁（Collitin）加到含0.1g茚三酮的50ml无水乙醇中。

（2）溶液Ⅱ：0.5g硝酸铜溶于50ml无水乙醇中。

（3）喷雾剂：使用前，将溶液Ⅰ和Ⅱ以50∶3之比例混合，喷后将薄层板放置在一块热板上直到颜色展现为止。在透过光线之后，可见到色泽逐渐增强，有些氨基酸首先出现色斑，根据不同氨基酸形成色斑的速度不同，利用铅笔及时标记就可以检测互相重叠的成分，许多氨基酸呈现特殊颜色。

3. 茚三酮－乙酸铬 1g茚三酮、2.5g乙酸铬〔Cd（AC）$_2$〕和10ml 冰醋酸溶于490ml甲醇中，喷后烘箱中于120℃加热，用于检定氨基酸。

4. 茚三酮－可力丁试剂 0.2～0.3g茚三酮溶于95ml水饱和的异丙醇或丁醇溶液中，加5ml可力丁（2，4，6－三甲基吡啶），喷后80～90℃加热30～60分钟，氨基酸显蓝色斑。

5. 去氢抗坏血酸 0.1g去氢抗坏血酸溶于5ml 60℃水中，用丁醇稀至100ml，喷雾后100℃加热5分钟，羟脯氨酸显淡紫蓝斑（25μg）；其他氨基酸显粉红到红斑（1～3μg）。

6. 重氮化试剂 把对氨基苯甲酸的盐酸（2%～3%）饱和溶液和5%亚硝酸钠溶液等体积混合后喷雾，再立即喷1M 1N氢氧化钠溶液，当酪氨酸、组氨酸存在时呈红橙色。

7. 重氮化对氨基苯磺酸试剂 对氨基苯磺酸4.5g加热溶于12M盐酸溶液45ml中，用水稀释至500ml，取稀释液10ml于冰浴中冷却后加入冷却的4.5%亚硝酸钠水溶液10ml，此试剂于0℃保留15分钟（低温时可稳定1～3天）。喷前加等体积的7%碳酸钠水溶液。

8. 对－二甲氨基苯甲醛－盐酸试剂 将2g对－二甲氨基苯甲醛溶于100ml 20%盐酸中，以此溶液喷滤纸后，于60℃加热干燥，当色氨酸及其衍生物存在时出现紫色斑点。

十、强心苷

1. 3，5－二硝基苯甲酸

（1）喷雾剂Ⅰ 将1g 3，5－二硝基苯甲酸溶于50ml甲醇和50ml 2M氢氧化钾混合液中。

（2）喷雾剂Ⅱ 2%3，5－二硝基苯甲酸甲醇溶液。

（3）喷雾剂Ⅲ 5.7%氢氧化钾醇液，薄层板先用Ⅱ轻轻喷之，再喷过量的Ⅲ，可得蓝～紫色斑点。

注：喷雾剂Ⅰ应单独使用。

2. 碱性苦味酸试剂 9ml 1%苦味酸乙醇溶液与1ml 10%氢氧化钠混匀即可，临用鲜配。

3. 亚硝酰铁氰化钠（硝普钠）－氢氧化钠试剂　1g 亚硝酰铁氰化钠溶于 100ml 2M 氢氧化钠－乙醇（1∶1）溶液，可作显色剂用，若作一般试管检识用，则需先加 0.3% 亚硝酰铁氰化钠溶液，再加 10% 氢氧化钠溶液即可。

4. 间二硝基苯试剂

（1）喷雾剂Ⅰ　10% 间二硝基苯的苯溶液。

（2）喷雾剂 Ⅱ　6g 氢氧化钠溶于 25ml 水中，再加 45ml 甲醇。

方法：先喷Ⅰ，于 60℃ 干燥后，再喷Ⅱ，强心苷显紫斑后变蓝并褪去，对于甲酰胺浸过的薄层板，喷雾前当于 60℃ 烘干。

5. 氯胺 T－三氯醋酸（Chlormine T－trichloroacetic acid）

（1）溶液Ⅰ　为新鲜制备的 3% 氯氨 T 水溶液。

（2）溶液Ⅱ　为 25% 三氯醋酸的乙醇液（可保存几天）

方法：临用前把 10ml Ⅰ液与 40ml Ⅱ液混合，喷后于 110℃ 加热 7 分钟，对于洋地黄苷在长波紫外光下可观察到蓝或黄色荧光。

6. 2，4，6－三硝基苯甲酸

（1）喷雾剂Ⅰ　为 0.1%2，4，6－三硝基苯甲酸的水－二甲基甲酰胺水溶液。

（2）喷雾剂Ⅱ　为 5% 碳酸钠水溶液。

（3）喷雾剂Ⅲ　为 5% 磷酸二氢钠溶液。

方法：薄层板分别以喷雾剂Ⅰ、Ⅱ喷后，在 90～100℃ 加热 4～5 分钟，放冷，最后喷以Ⅲ，强心苷呈橙～红色斑点。

十一、有机酸类

1. 溴酚蓝试剂

（1）0.1g 溴酚蓝溶解在 5ml 乙醇中，再与 3ml 0.05M 氢氧化钠和 20ml 水混合。

（2）0.04% 溴酚蓝乙醇溶液，用 0.1M 氢氧化钠调至微碱性即可。

2. 溴甲酚绿（蓝）指示剂　溴甲酚绿 0.04g 溶于乙醇 100ml，加 0.1M 氢氧化钠溶液至兰色刚出现，喷后在兰色背景上显黄色，如果展开剂中含乙酸，则在喷雾前将薄层在 120℃ 烘烤除去。

3. 溴甲酚紫（红）指示剂　溴甲酚紫 0.04g 溶于 50% 乙醇 500ml 中，用 0.1M 氢氧化钠溶液调至 pH 10.0，喷前薄层在 100℃ 烤 10 分钟，冷至室温后喷显色剂，有机酸存在时，则在兰色背景上显黄色。

4. 百里酚酞碱溶液　百里酚酞 50mg 溶于 2% 氢氧化钠溶液 100ml，喷后在灰或兰色背景上显白色斑点。

5. 联苯胺－亚硝酸钠试剂

（1）溶液Ⅰ　联苯胺 2.5g 溶于浓盐酸 7ml 及水 500ml 。

（2）溶液Ⅱ　10% 亚硝酸钠溶液。

方法：临用前将 Ⅰ与 Ⅱ以 3∶2 混合，喷后于紫外灯下 254nm 观察荧光，用于检测有机酸类。

6. 2，6－二氯苯酚－靛酚钠盐　为 0.1% 2，6－二氯苯酚－靛酚钠盐的乙醇溶液。

喷后稍加热后，在兰色背景上可呈现红色斑点，用于检测有机酸酮酸。

7. 吖啶试剂 为0.05%吖啶的乙醇溶液，用于检测苹果酸等。

十二、其他类化合物

1. 硫酸肼 取硫酸肼饱和的水溶液90ml同10ml 4M盐酸溶液混合，将湿层析谱分别在暴置于氨蒸气前后于长波紫外灯下检视之，用于检测胡椒酰、香草醛及乙基香草醛。

2. 偏高碘酸钠-联苯胺

（1）喷雾剂Ⅰ 为0.1%偏高碘酸钠的水溶液。

（2）喷雾剂Ⅱ 将1.8g联苯胺溶于50ml 0.2M盐酸。

先喷Ⅰ，5分钟后再喷Ⅱ，含1，2-二醇基（糖、多元醇）的化合物在蓝色背景可出现白色斑点。

3. 四乙基铅 以1%四乙基铅的苯溶液喷雾，喷后于110℃加热5分钟，1，2-二醇基化合物在棕色背景下呈白色斑点。

4. 乙二胺 将乙二胺与等体积的水或稀氢氧化钠混合即得。喷后于50~60℃加热20分钟，与短波或长波紫外灯下检查，用于检测儿茶酚胺类化合物。

5. 氯化铜试剂 以0.5%氯化铜的水溶液喷雾。β-肟络合物在喷后立即呈绿色，α-肟络合物则于喷雾后在110℃ 加热10分钟后才生成棕绿色的斑点。

6. 甲醛-硫酸 将0.2ml 37%甲醛溶液溶于10ml浓硫酸中，展开后之薄层板立即用喷雾剂喷之，用于检测多环芳香族化合物，不同的芳香族化合物可产生不同的颜色。也可用于生物碱的测定。

7. 铁氰化钾

（1）溶液Ⅰ：1%铁氰化钾水溶液。

（2）溶液Ⅱ：15%氢氧化钠溶液。

（3）喷雾剂：取1.5ml溶液Ⅰ，以20ml水稀释之，加10ml溶液Ⅱ即得。喷后于长波紫外灯下观察，用于检测维生素B（硫胺反应）。

8. 硝普钠-氢氧化钠 配制见十.3，对于甲基铜，活性亚甲基的化合物呈红紫色斑点。

9. 羟胺-氯化铁

（1）溶液Ⅰ 将20g氯化羟基胺（盐酸羟胺）溶于50ml水中，加乙醇稀释至200ml，存放于冷处。

（2）溶液Ⅱ 将50g氢氧化钾溶于最少量的水中，用乙醇稀释至500ml。

（3）喷雾剂Ⅰ 将溶液Ⅰ与Ⅱ以1:2之比混合，并把氢氧化钾沉淀滤去，所得最终溶液应保存于冰箱中，此液约可稳定2周。

（4）喷雾剂Ⅱ 将10g氯化铁（$FeCl_3 \cdot 6H_2O$）细粉溶于20ml 36%盐酸中，此液用20ml乙醚共同振摇直至成均匀溶液为止，此溶液在密闭容器中可保存较长时间。

方法：层析谱先以喷雾剂Ⅰ喷之，在室温稍干燥后，再以Ⅱ喷之。

10. 硝酸银-高锰酸钾

（1）溶液Ⅰ：临用前将0.1M硝酸银，2M 2N氢氧化铵和2N氢氧化钠以1:1:2之比混合即得。

（2）溶液Ⅱ：将0.5g高锰酸钾和1g碳酸钠溶于100ml中即得。

（3）喷雾剂：将等体积的Ⅰ、Ⅱ混合，因本试剂不稳定，应于临用前鲜配，喷后还原性物质在蓝～绿色背景上可出现淡黄色斑点。

11. 硝酸银－氢氧化铵 0.1M 0.1N硝酸银与5N氢氧化铵于临用前按1∶5混合即得（注意久置会生成叠氮化银爆炸物）。喷后于105℃加热5～10分钟，至暗黑色变至最深为止，用于检测还原性化合物。

12. 磷钼酸试剂 喷后于120℃加热直至形成最佳色斑为止，用于检测还原性合物、类脂、甾醇及甾体化合物。

13. 硫酸－硝酸铈铁 为含1%硝酸铈铵的50%硫酸溶液，喷后于105℃烘10分钟至显色，用于检测鬼臼毒素类化合物等。

14. 4－羟基苯甲醛－硫酸

（1）溶液Ⅰ 50%硫酸。

（2）溶液Ⅱ 2%4－羟基苯甲醛的甲醇溶液。

（3）喷雾剂 使用前将溶液Ⅰ 5ml与溶液Ⅱ 50ml充分混合，喷后于105℃加热3～4分钟或于60℃加热10分钟，皂苷元、皮质甾体（α位末取代的3－甾酮类化合物）应产生黄～粉红色斑点。

15. 斯托克试剂 溶解30g硫酸亚铁（$FeSO_4$）和20g酒石酸于水中，稀释至1L，在临用前加浓氨水直至沉淀刚出现又重新溶解为止。

16. 碘化钾－碘化汞 溶解50g碘化钾于500ml水中，再以碘化汞使之饱和（约需120g）。用前稀释即可。

（许翔鸿）